BASIC GUIDE TO
DENTAL INSTRUMENTS

BASIC GUIDE TO DENTAL INSTRUMENTS

Second Edition

Carmen Scheller-Sheridan

C.D.A., R.D.N., Dip. Ad. Ed., M.A. O.D.E.
Lecturer in Dental Nursing
Dublin Dental University Hospital
Trinity College Dublin
Republic of Ireland

WILEY-BLACKWELL

A John Wiley & Sons, Ltd., Publication

This edition first published 2011
© 2006 by Blackwell Publishing Ltd
© 2011 by Carmen Scheller-Sheridan

Wiley-Blackwell is an imprint of John Wiley & Sons, formed by the merger of Wiley's global Scientific, Technical and Medical business with Blackwell Publishing.

Registered office: John Wiley & Sons, Ltd, The Atrium, Southern Gate, Chichester, West Sussex, PO19 8SQ, UK

Editorial offices: 9600 Garsington Road, Oxford, OX4 2DQ, UK
The Atrium, Southern Gate, Chichester, West Sussex, PO19 8SQ, UK
2121 State Avenue, Ames, Iowa 50014-8300, USA

For details of our global editorial offices, for customer services and for information about how to apply for permission to reuse the copyright material in this book please see our website at www.wiley.com/wiley-blackwell.

The right of the author to be identified as the author of this work has been asserted in accordance with the UK Copyright, Designs and Patents Act 1988.

Library of Congress Cataloging-in-Publication Data

Scheller-Sheridan, Carmen.
  Basic guide to dental instruments / Carmen Scheller-Sheridan. – 2nd ed.
      p. ; cm.
  Includes bibliographical references and index.
  ISBN-13: 978-1-4443-3532-3 (pbk.)
  ISBN-10: 1-4443-3532-4 (pbk.)
  1. Dental instruments and apparatus–Handbooks, manuals, etc.   I. Title.
  [DNLM: 1. Dental Instruments–Handbooks.   WU 49]
  RK681.S33 2011
  617.6′0028–dc23

                                                        2011021940

A catalogue record for this book is available from the British Library.

Set in 9/11.5pt Sabon by Aptara® Inc., New Delhi, India
Printed and bound by CPI Group (UK) Ltd, Croydon, CR0 4YY

C9781444335323_190724

CONTENTS

To my dear husband, Padraig, and sweet daughter, Abigail,
for all of their love and support.

ACKNOWLEDGEMENTS

I would like to thank the many people who supported me with this publication: Professor Noel Claffey, Professor June Nunn, Tina Gorman, Joan Brennan, Madonna Bell, Pascaline Fresneau, Una Lannon and Helen Phipps. Thank you to Dr Declan Furlong who provided me with some images and to Mr Mark Thompson for photographing many of the dental instruments.

Thank you to the following companies and people who supplied photographs:

American Eagle Instruments Inc.
Biomet 3i
DENTSPLY Ash® Instruments
Dr Declan Furlong
Dynaflex
Garrison Dental Solutions
Henry Schein Ireland
Hu-Friedy
J. Morita Europe GMBH
Kerr
Kodak
Laerdal Medical Ltd
Learning and Teaching Scotland
LM – Instruments Oy
L&R Manufacturing
Dr Anthony Maganzini
Integra LifeSciences Corporation, Plainsboro, NJ
Ormco Europe
Owandy Dental Imaging
Premier Dental Products Company
Dr Frank Quinn
Roydent Dental Products
SDI
Septodont
Sirona Dental Systems
Sybron Endo
Total Care
Ultrasonics
W&H (UK) LTD
Young Dental

HOW TO USE THIS BOOK

As the dental profession evolves, there is an increasing demand for supplementary material that can keep up with advancing trends. 'Hands on' practical experience is essential for anyone in the dental profession, and this needs to be supplemented with written information to reinforce our practical experiences.

This illustrated manual has been prepared for students working and studying in the dental profession. It may be used as a study aid or kept in the dental surgery as a reference guide. This manual is intended to complement other methods of learning, i.e. textbooks, lecture notes, etc., and is not meant to be a comprehensive resource.

Because many dental instruments look similar, and can be confusing to a student, the 'false friends' sub-sections identify instruments that may resemble the particular instrument. This manual is not intended to be a complete representation of all dental instruments, but it does include examples from each dental discipline. As many dental instruments are multi-functional and are referred to by more than one name, where possible, these are given beside the name of the instrument. Complete set-ups have been included at the end of most sections for various procedures. The dental professional may have to modify these lists depending on the operator's preference.

Each section is dedicated to a specific discipline or division of dentistry. Some instruments feature in many sections, and these have been included in the set-up sub-sections of the relevant sections. Infection control is a fundamental requirement in the dental surgery, and as such the first section is dedicated to this area. This section aims to introduce the principles of health and safety, which must always be at the forefront of a dental professional's mind. Contact the legislative bodies for appropriate regulations and legislation relevant to your workplace.

The instruments in this guide are not to scale, and during photography some colours may have been altered.

SECTION 1
INFECTION CONTROL IN THE DENTAL SURGERY

It is the responsibility of the dental team to ensure that the appropriate and correct procedures are carried out in relation to infection control to protect the patients, the public and themselves.

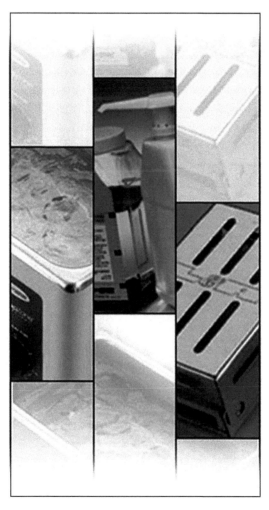

Basic Guide to Dental Instruments, Second Edition. Carmen Scheller-Sheridan.
© 2011 Carmen Scheller-Sheridan. Published 2011 by Blackwell Publishing Ltd.

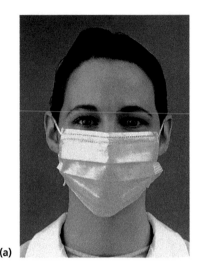

(a)

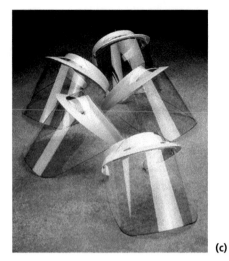

(c)

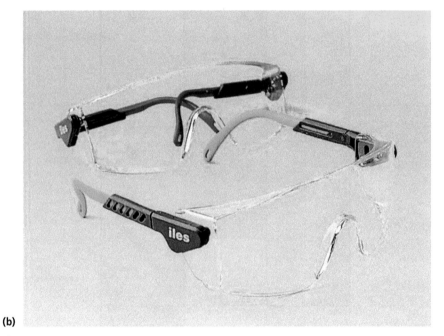

(b)

Figure 1.1

PROTECTIVE WEAR

FIGURE 1.1a, b, c

Name
(a) Mask (b) Safety glasses (c) Face shields

Function, precautions and directions for use
- To protect the dental team from micro-organisms, debris, splatter and chemicals
- A mask is worn to protect the mucous membranes of the nose and mouth. It filters out small particles
  - Should always be changed between each patient or before if it is visibly soiled
  - Should be worn during patient care, sterilisation, disinfection, cleaning procedures and during laboratory work
- Safety glasses and/or face shields are worn to protect the mucous membranes of the eyes
  - Should be disinfected between patients
  - A face shield can be used instead of safety glasses, but a mask must still be worn
  - Should be large enough to cover the eye area completely and provide protection from the top and side. With some safety glasses additional top and side shields have to be added to be used for this purpose
  - Safety glasses are available to fit over prescription eye wear
  - Must be shatterproof

Varieties
Different types of masks and glasses available

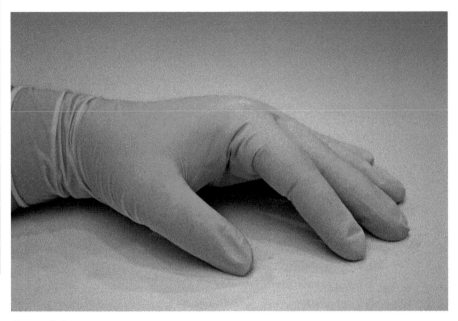

Figure 1.2

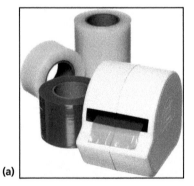

(a)

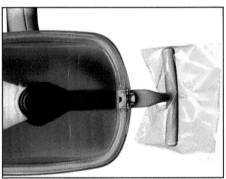

(b)

Figure 1.3

FIGURE 1.2

Name
Protective gloves

Function and directions for use
- To protect the dental team from direct contact with micro-organisms, debris, splatter and chemicals
- Worn during patient care when coming in contact with contaminated objects and chemicals, and when working intra-orally
- Always change between patients
- Do not wash gloves
- Replace damaged and ripped gloves immediately
- Always wash and dry hands thoroughly prior to donning gloves
- It is important to make sure gloves fit properly

Varieties
- Made from many different materials, i.e. latex, vinyl and nitrile
- Available packaged as sterile surgical gloves
- Rubber utility gloves/heavy duty gloves are used during sterilisation procedures

WORK SURFACES

FIGURE 1.3a, b

Name
Non-permeable barriers

Function and features
- Used to cover surfaces to prevent contamination
- Must be impermeable
- Single use; to be disposed of in the contaminated waste

Varieties
Many different types and sizes available

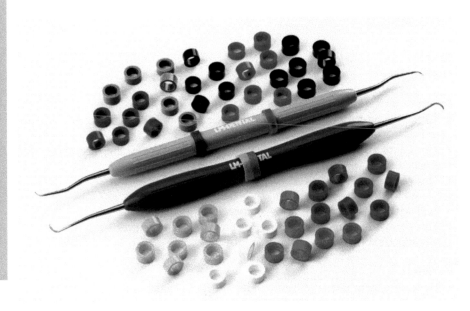

Figure 1.4

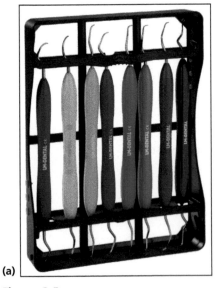

(a)

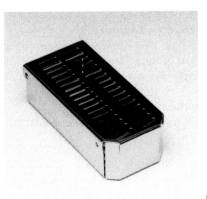

(b)

Figure 1.5

ITEMS USED FOR IDENTIFICATION AND ORGANISATION DURING STERILISATION

FIGURE 1.4

Name
Coloured identification rings

Function and feature
- Used to organise and identify instruments
- Autoclavable

Varieties
- Many different types and sizes available
- Coloured autoclavable tape can also be used

FIGURE 1.5a, b, c

Name
Instrument cassettes

Function(s)
- Used to organise and identify instruments during sterilisation and disinfection
- Can double as an instrument tray during procedures

Varieties
Many different types and sizes available, including plastic and metal types

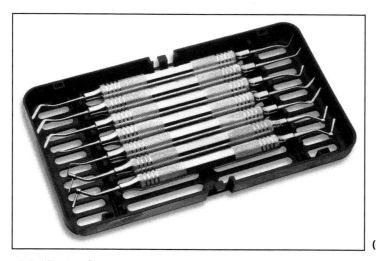

(c)

Figure 1.5 (*Continued*)

INFECTION CONTROL IN
THE DENTAL SURGERY

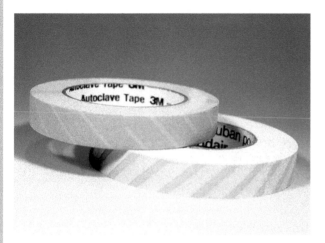

Figure 1.6

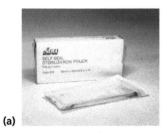

(a)

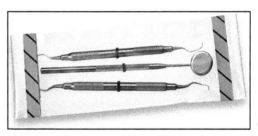

(b)

Figure 1.7

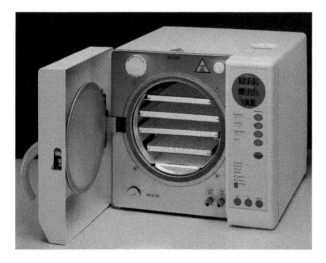

Figure 1.8

FIGURE 1.6

Name
Autoclave tape

Function and features
- Used to secure instrument wrap or pouches prior to sterilisation
- Will change colour once exposed to a certain temperature, but this does not indicate whether sterilisation has occurred
- Can be written on to indicate the contents of the package

Varieties
Many different types and sizes available

FIGURE 1.7a, b

Name
Sterilisation pouch

Functions and features
- Used to wrap instruments prior to sterilisation
- Aids in organisation of instruments
- One side may be transparent to allow for viewing of the pouch contents (Figure 1.7a, b)
- Coloured markings indicate that a certain temperature has been reached during the sterilisation cycle
- Instruments will remain sterile in pouch until it is punctured or opened

Varieties
Many different types and sizes available

STERILISATION EQUIPMENT

FIGURE 1.8

Name
Autoclave

Function and directions for use
- Uses steam under high pressure to achieve sterilisation
- Follow manufacturer's directions for use
- Consult local legislation and guidelines in regard to appropriate sterilisation procedures

Varieties
Many different types and sizes available

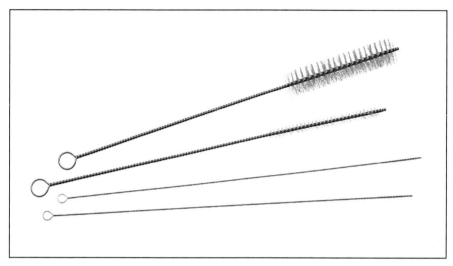

Figure 1.9

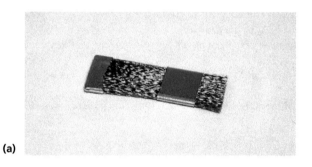

(a)

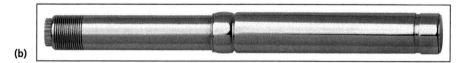

(b)

Figure 1.10

MANUAL CLEANING AIDS

FIGURE 1.9

Name

Bottle brushes

Functions, features and precautions
- Manual cleaning is never recommended except when ultrasonic cleaning is not effective in removing debris
- Used along with a soapy cleaner to remove debris prior to sterilisation
- Allows cleaning inside suction tubes
- Long handle allows a greater distance between the operator and the contaminated object
- Should always be used submersed in water to reduce splatter
- Always wear heavy duty utility gloves while using bottle brushes

Varieties

Many different types and sizes available

FIGURE 1.10a, b

Name

Bur brushes

Function and precautions
- Manual cleaning is only recommended when ultrasonic cleaning is not effective in removing debris
- Used along with cleaner to remove debris prior to sterilisation
- Allows for the cleaning of burs with small, hard-to-clean flutes
- Always wear rubber utility gloves/heavy duty gloves while using bur brushes

Varieties

Many different types and sizes available

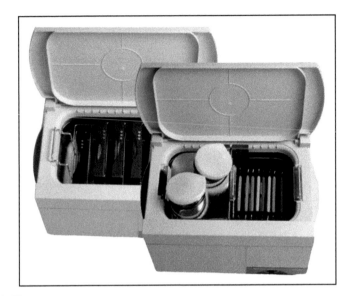

Figure 1.11

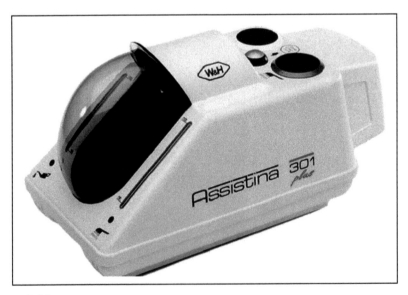

Figure 1.12

FIGURE 1.11

Name

Ultrasonic cleaner

Function(s) and directions for use

- Used along with a soapy cleaner
- Uses sound waves to reduce bioburden and debris from instruments prior to sterilisation
- Follow manufacturer's instructions for solution types and length of time needed for cleaning

Varieties

Many different types and sizes available

FIGURE 1.12

Name

Assistina

Function(s) and directions for use

- Uses air to run cleaning fluid solution and oil through handpieces
- Used to expel debris from handpieces
- Plastic cover over handpiece attachment is used to reduce aerosol
- Follow manufacturer's instructions for use

Varieties

Many different types available

INFECTION CONTROL IN
THE DENTAL SURGERY

SECTION 2
DENTAL RADIOGRAPHY

Radiographs are important tools in the diagnosing of dental disease. There are many types of radiographs available, all of which are used for different purposes. There are two main types of dental radiographic films: intra-oral and extra-oral.

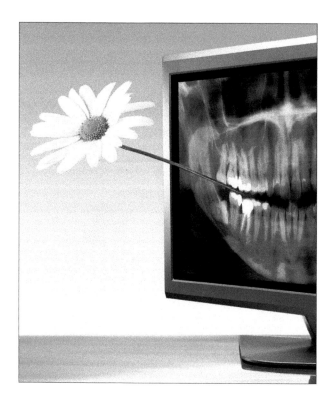

Basic Guide to Dental Instruments, Second Edition. Carmen Scheller-Sheridan.
© 2011 Carmen Scheller-Sheridan. Published 2011 by Blackwell Publishing Ltd.

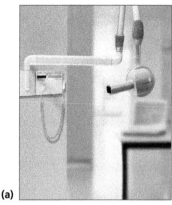

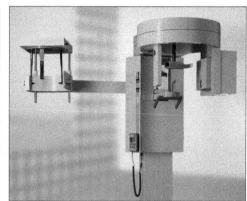

(a)   (b)

Figure 2.1

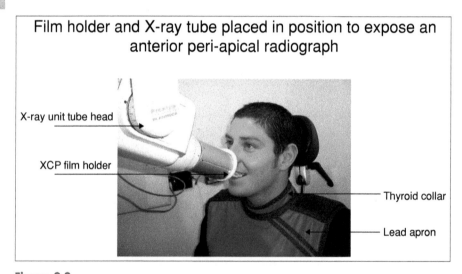

Film holder and X-ray tube placed in position to expose an anterior peri-apical radiograph

X-ray unit tube head

XCP film holder

Thyroid collar

Lead apron

Figure 2.2

FIGURE 2.1a, b

Name
(a) Intra-oral X-ray machine (b) Extra-oral X-ray machine

Functions
- Intra-oral X-ray machines are used for exposing occlusal, peri-apical and bite-wing radiographs
- Extra-oral X-ray machines are used for exposing panoramic/OPG (orthopantomograph) radiographs and cephalometric radiographs

Varieties
Machines from different manufacturers may vary in design

FIGURE 2.2

Name
Lead apron and thyroid collar

Function and precautions
- A lead apron and thyroid collar must be used to protect the patient from radiation during X-ray procedures
- The lead apron is used with a thyroid collar that must cover the radio-sensitive tissues (from the thyroid downwards and including the lap area)
- The lead apron must be hung up, not folded because folding the apron will cause the lead inside to crack, causing radiation to pass through

Varieties
Different styles available from various manufacturers

DENTAL RADIOGRAPHY

DENTAL RADIOGRAPHY

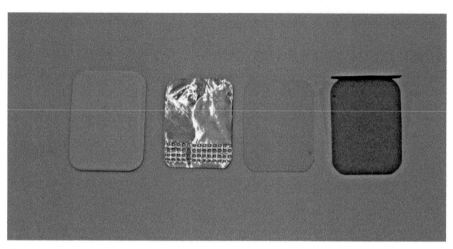

Figure 2.3

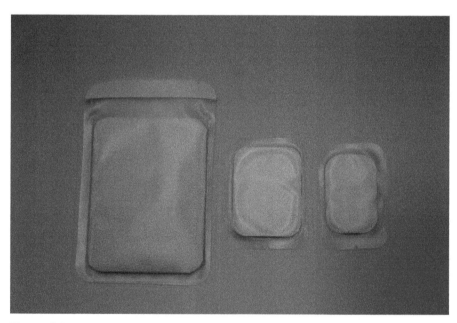

Figure 2.4

CONVENTIONAL INTRA-ORAL RADIOGRAPH FILM

FIGURES 2.3; 2.4

- A detailed radiograph film, which is exposed while in the patient's mouth
- Used in conjunction with a film holder for accurate placement
- Some films may be covered in a clear plastic sleeve for infection control and prevention purposes (see Figure 2.4)
- Every film has a bump to assist in film orientation
- The bump always faces towards the X-ray tube
- Inside the film packet:
  - Black paper on either side of film to protect film from light (see Figure 2.3)
  - On the back of the film there is a thin sheet of lead foil to absorb stray/scatter radiation

DENTAL RADIOGRAPHY

DENTAL RADIOGRAPHY

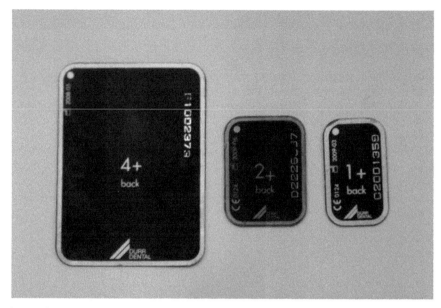

Figure 2.5

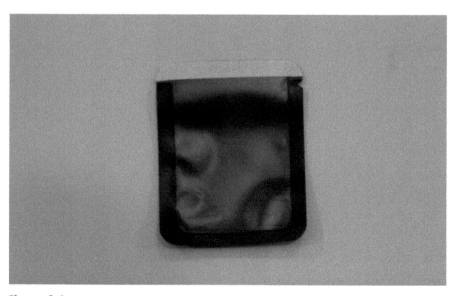

Figure 2.6

INDIRECT DIGITAL RADIOGRAPH FILM – PHOSPHOR PLATES

FIGURES 2.5; 2.6

- Phosphor plates are thinner than digital sensors and can be used with the extension cone paralleling (XCP) holders
- After exposure using a phosphor plate it is loaded into a scanner allows the operator to view the radiograph digitally
- Once the image is produced the phosphor plate is 'wiped clean' for reuse using a single use plastic sleeve for infection control and prevention
- A detailed radiograph film, which is exposed while in the patient's mouth
- Used in conjunction with a film holder for accurate placement
- Phosphor plates are always covered in a plastic sleeve for infection prevention purposes (Figure 2.6)
- Every film has a bump to assist in film orientation
- The bump always faces towards the X-ray tube

DENTAL RADIOGRAPHY

DENTAL RADIOGRAPHY

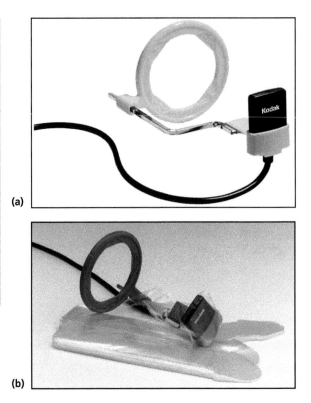

(a)

(b)

Figure 2.7

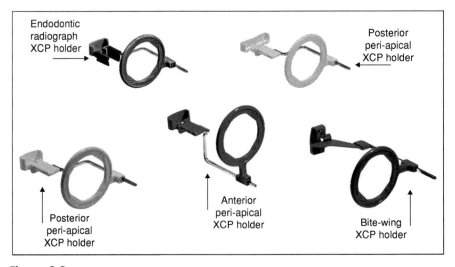

Endodontic radiograph XCP holder

Posterior peri-apical XCP holder

Posterior peri-apical XCP holder

Anterior peri-apical XCP holder

Bite-wing XCP holder

Figure 2.8

FIGURE 2.7a, b

Name
Digital radiography aids: (a) Digital Sensor in an XCP film holder (b) Barrier wrapped around sensor and XCP film holder

Functions
- A way to produce a filmless radiographic image
- A sensor is used instead of a film
- As sensors cannot be sterilised, a non-permeable barrier must be placed over the sensor and XCP film holder (see Figure 2.7b and Section 1)

The digital radiographical image is viewed on a computer screen and stored in the computer. It is easily retrieved.

Varieties
There are many manufacturers of digital radiography equipment

RADIOGRAPHIC ACCESSORIES AND EQUIPMENT

FIGURE 2.8

Name
XCP film holders

Functions
- To aid in film placement for intra-oral radiographs
- The holders shown in Figure 2.8 are for use with digital radiography; the holders for ordinary radiographic films are similar
- These XCP film holders are used with the paralleling technique
- A film holder helps to take the most accurate radiograph possible, reducing radiation exposure through retakes

Note: It is the duty of the dental team to minimise the amount of radiation exposure to the patient

Varieties
- Different film holders are available depending on the type of radiograph indicated and operator preference (e.g. styrofoam bite block, digital radiograph holders and Snap-A-Ray instrument)
- Check legislation and local rules in your area to identify which film holders are acceptable

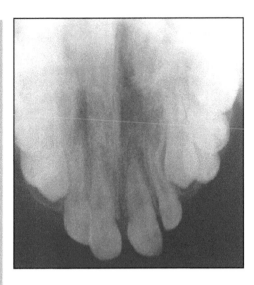

Figure 2.9

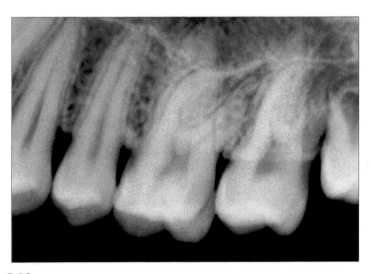

Figure 2.10

FIGURE 2.9

Name
Occlusal radiograph

Type
Intra-oral radiograph

Functions
- Provides an image of the maxillary or mandibular arch
- Used to check eruption of teeth, to locate foreign objects, jaw fractures and supernumerary teeth, and to detect hard and soft tissue abnormalities

FIGURE 2.10

Name
Peri-apical radiograph

Type
Intra-oral radiograph

Functions
- Provides an image of the entire tooth (crown to root and supporting structures)
- A detailed image of two to four teeth may be obtained on one radiograph
- Used to show apical infections, retained roots, morphology of roots, length of root canal, post-trauma, apical cysts, and evaluation of implants, lesions and periodontal status

Varieties
- Different sizes of films are available depending on the patient's mouth size and tolerance level
- The same size of radiographic film can be used for bite-wing radiographs

DENTAL RADIOGRAPHY

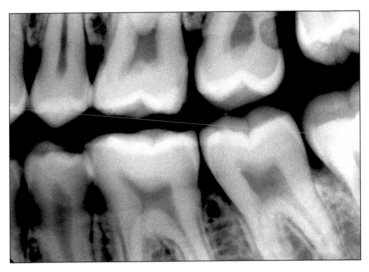

Figure 2.11

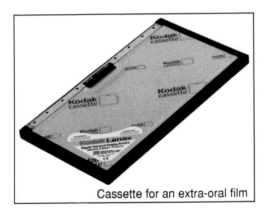

Cassette for an extra-oral film   **Figure 2.12**

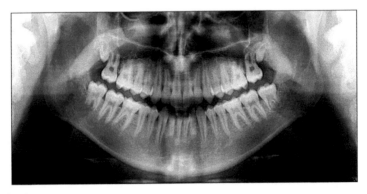

Figure 2.13

FIGURE 2.11

Name
Bite-wing radiograph

Type
Intra-oral radiograph

Functions
- Provides an image of the crowns of the premolars and molars on either the right or the left side
- Used to detect interproximal caries, recurrent caries and to check bone levels

Varieties
- The same size of radiographic film can be used for peri-apical radiographs
- Can have vertical and horizontal bite-wing radiographs

EXTRA-ORAL RADIOGRAPHS

FIGURE 2.12

- Are exposed outside the patient's mouth
- Panoramic radiograph film is placed within the cassette, then on the panoramic X-ray machine
- Will show a full view of the maxillary and mandibular dental arches, but with less detail than an intra-oral radiograph
- The film is protected from light in the cassette, which is held between two intensifying screens (see Figure 2.12)
- This type of film needs a special machine for exposure

FIGURE 2.13

Name
Panoramic radiograph/OPG

Type
Extra-oral radiograph

Functions
- Provides an image of all the teeth in both the maxillary and mandibular arches and supporting structures
- Used to view the periodontium, bone levels, pathology, temporomandibular joints, sinuses, impacted teeth, position of dental nerves, eruption patterns, orientation of third molars, retained roots, fractures, cysts and restorations

DENTAL RADIOGRAPHY

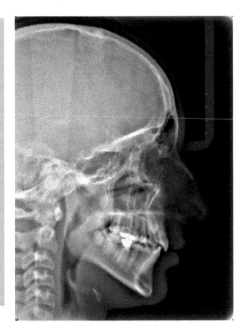

Figure 2.14

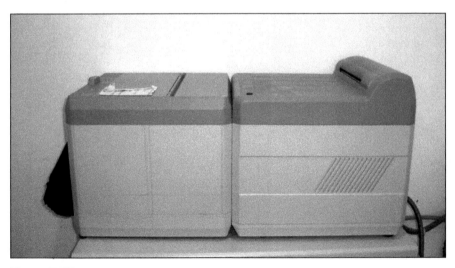

Figure 2.15

FIGURE 2.14

Name
Cephalometric radiograph

Type
Extra-oral radiograph

Functions
- Provides an image of the skull – mostly used in orthodontic assessments and oral surgery
- Allows the operator to take measurements of the skull
- Used to monitor treatment progression and to detect fractures

FIGURE 2.15

Name
Automatic processor

Function and precautions
- Film processing includes the steps taken to make a latent (non-visible) image visible
- The automatic processor shields the radiograph from light, which can cause artefacts and adversely affect processing while the rollers carry the film through the solutions and the dryer
- Developer and fixer chemicals are contained within the automatic processor and should be handled wearing protective equipment
- Follow the manufacturer's instructions for use of the processor
- Dispose of chemicals according to your local health and safety guidelines

Varieties
- Radiographs are transported through the processor usually by rollers or conveyors
- Radiographs can be processed by the manual method

> **!** *The following items relate to health and safety in radiography. Check local legislation and guidelines in your area, as these differ between countries.*

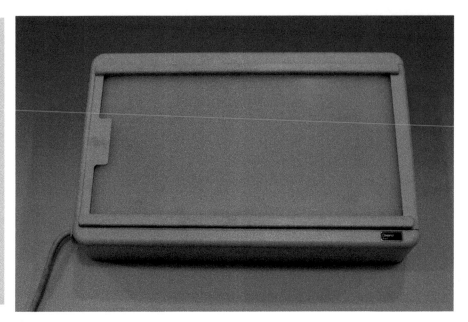

Figure 2.16

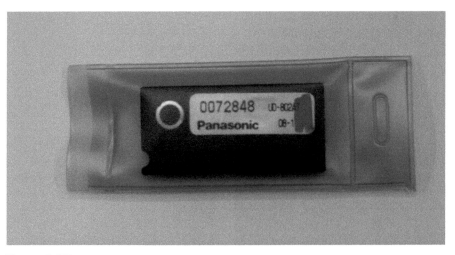

Figure 2.17

FIGURE 2.16

Name
X-ray viewer

Function and labelling of films
- Used with a light source to view patient radiographs
- All radiographs must be placed in film mounts and labelled with the patient's name, date, operator's name and chart number (if applicable)

Varieties
Many varieties of X-ray viewers and film mounts are available from different manufacturers

FIGURE 2.17

Name
Dosimeter/radiation monitoring badge

Function and directions for use
- Used to measure level of radiation received by an individual
- Monitored by local radiological board
- Aids in quality assurance process by monitoring safety of X-ray units
- Badge needs to be worn around the hip area and sent back to the radiological board to read dosage levels
- Each individual should be allocated their own dosimeter/radiation monitoring badge, as each individual needs to know their own dosage level

DENTAL RADIOGRAPHY

SECTION 3
BASIC INSTRUMENTS

There are a few basic instruments that are universal to almost every procedure in dentistry.

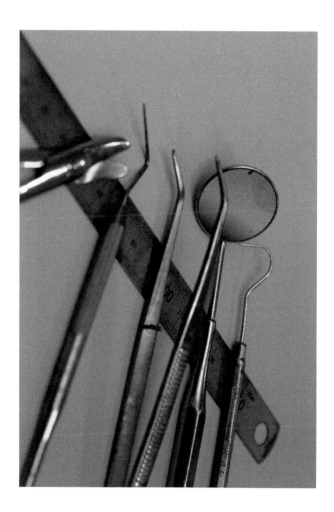

Basic Guide to Dental Instruments, Second Edition. Carmen Scheller-Sheridan.
© 2011 Carmen Scheller-Sheridan. Published 2011 by Blackwell Publishing Ltd.

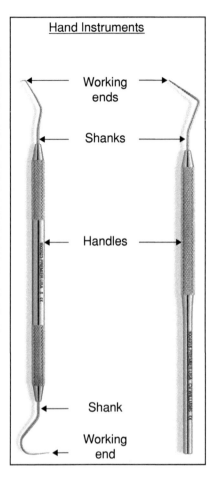

Hand Instruments

Working ends

Shanks

Handles

Shank

Working end

Figure 3.1

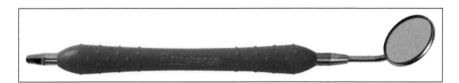

Figure 3.2

GENERAL FEATURES OF DENTAL INSTRUMENTS

FIGURE 3.1

Working end(s) of instruments
- Are the functional parts of the instrument
- Can have a variety of functions including cutting, packing, carving, placing and condensing
- Are adapted to the function of the particular instrument
- May be bevelled (i.e. the working end is cut at an angle)
- An instrument can be single-ended (one working end) or double-ended (two working ends)

Shank of an instrument
- The part between the working end and the handle
- Can be straight or angled
- The function of the instrument determines the angle and flexibility of the shank

Handle of an instrument
- Is the part of the instrument that the operator grasps
- Provides stability and leverage
- Design is related to the function of the instrument
- Examples:
  - The handle of an upper extraction forceps may be curved to facilitate a palm grasp for the operator
  - The handle of a rubber dam clamp forceps is rounded to fit in the palm of the operator's hand
  - A serrated handle allows a better grip
  - A large handle allows a palm grasp

THE BASIC DENTAL INSTRUMENTS

FIGURE 3.2

Name
Mouth mirror and handle

Functions
- To provide indirect vision
- To reflect light
- For retraction and protection of oral tissues
- For magnification (the number of the mirror represents size of mirror head)

Varieties
- Single-sided or double-sided
- Can be disposable
- Plain or magnifying

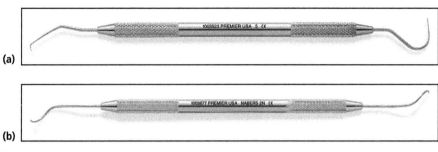

Figure 3.3

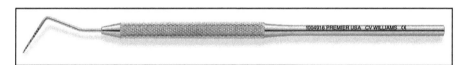

Figure 3.4

FIGURE 3.3a, b

Name
(a) Sickle/contra-angled probe (b) Nabers probe

Functions
- Detection of:
  - defective pits and fissures
  - calculus
  - deficient margins of restorations, crowns and bridges
  - caries
- Examination (pointed tip allows good tactile sensitivity)

Varieties
- Can be single-ended or double-ended
- Many different styles available
- Working ends may vary (straight, curved)

False friends
Periodontal probe, endodontic probe (DG16 probe), lateral condenser

FIGURE 3.4

Name
Periodontal probe

Function and features
- Measure the depth of periodontal pockets
- Tip is calibrated in millimetres
- Blunt end reduces the possibility of tissue trauma

Varieties
- Single-ended or double-ended
- Can be straight, curved or at right angles
- Plastic types available

False friends
Sickle/contra-angled probe/sickle probe, endodontic probe/DG16 probe and endodontic spreader

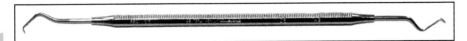

Figure 3.5

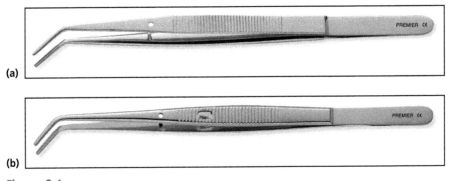

(a)

(b)

Figure 3.6

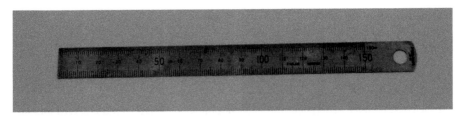

Figure 3.7

FIGURE 3.5

Name
Briault probe

Function and feature
- Detection of caries on mesial and distal surfaces
- The angled working ends facilitate adaptation to interproximal surfaces

False friend
Furcation probe

FIGURE 3.6a, b

Name
(a) College tweezers (b) Locking college tweezers

Functions
- Placing small objects in the mouth and retrieving small objects from the mouth
- Locking type 'lock' to prevent dropping materials

Varieties
- Locking and non-locking types
- Working ends can be straight, curved, serrated or smooth

False friends
Tissue dissecting forceps, toothed dissecting forceps

FIGURE 3.7

Name
Metal ruler

Function
Measurement of length, e.g. endodontic K files

Varieties
- Can be calibrated in different units of measure
- Plastic type available

BASIC INSTRUMENTS

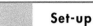

Set-up

Examination

- Mouth mirror and handle
- Sickle/contra-angled probe
- College tweezers

Optional: Briault probe, metal ruler and periodontal probe

SECTION 4

INSTRUMENTS AND SUNDRIES USED IN MOISTURE CONTROL

Properties of dental materials can be altered by moisture. The dental team can use specific instruments and sundries to aid in moisture control.

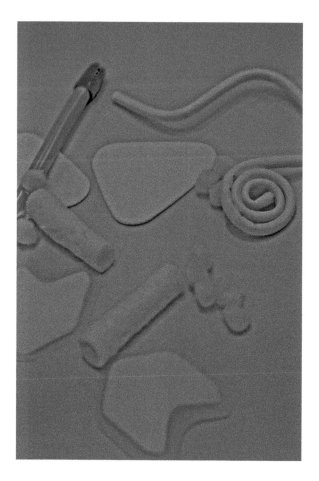

Basic Guide to Dental Instruments, Second Edition. Carmen Scheller-Sheridan.
© 2011 Carmen Scheller-Sheridan. Published 2011 by Blackwell Publishing Ltd.

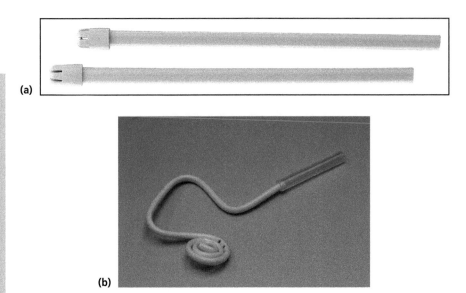

Figure 4.1

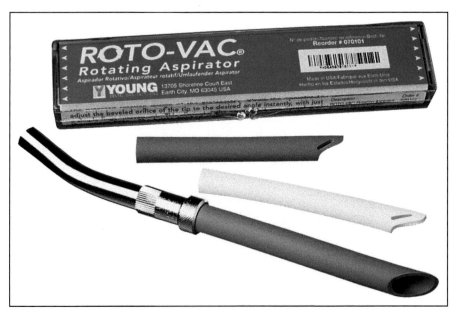

Figure 4.2

FIGURE 4.1a, b

Name
Disposable saliva ejector/low-volume suction

Function and features
- Low-volume evacuation of the mouth
- Tolerated easily by the patient
- Plastic types are single use and flexible – to suit clinical need

Varieties
- Metal or plastic
- Plastic ones come in a variety of colours and shapes and can be adapted for particular uses

FIGURE 4.2

Name
High-volume suction tip

Functions
- High-volume evacuation of the mouth
- Retraction and protection of tissues
- Reduction of aerosols created by handpieces

Varieties
- Metal (autoclavable), plastic (autoclavable or disposable – check manufacturer's instructions)
- Various lengths, shapes and sizes

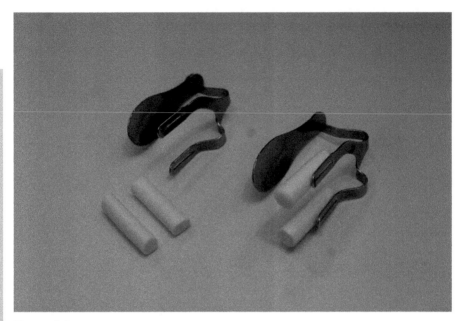

Figure 4.3

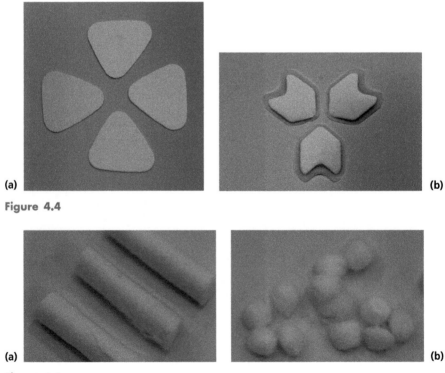

(a) (b)

Figure 4.4

(a) (b)

Figure 4.5

FIGURE 4.3

Name

Garmer cotton wool roll holders

Functions

- Moisture control
- Hold cotton rolls against the buccal and lingual surfaces (mandibular teeth)
- Retract cheek and tongue

Varieties

Separate holders for left and right sides

FIGURE 4.4a, b

Name

Disposable dry aid/dry guard

Functions and directions for use

- Moisture control
- Absorb excess saliva
- Place close to the opening of the parotid salivary duct

Varieties

Made from a variety of materials, e.g. cardboard or an absorbent material enclosed in a plastic cover

FIGURE 4.5a, b

Name

(a) Disposable cotton wool rolls (b) Cotton pellets

Functions

- Moisture control – absorb saliva, blood or excess dental materials
- Can be used to deliver materials to and from the mouth

Varieties

Various sizes available

INSTRUMENTS AND SUNDRIES USED IN
MOISTURE CONTROL

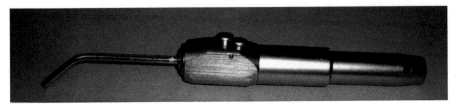

Figure 4.6

FIGURE 4.6

Name
Metal air/water syringe or referred to as 3-in-1 syringe

Functions and parts
- Provides spray of air, water or a combination of both
- Retraction
- Has a handle, controls and a tip (the tip can be of metal or plastic)

Varieties
- Different angled tips available for ease of access
- Can have plastic disposable tips for infection control purposes

INSTRUMENTS AND SUNDRIES USED IN
MOISTURE CONTROL

Set-up

Fissure sealants
- Mouth mirror and handle (p. 34, 35)
- Sickle/contra-angled probe (p. 36, 37)
- College tweezers (p. 39, 40)
- Disposable saliva ejector (p. 42, 43)
- Garmer cotton wool roll holders (mandibular sealants) (p. 44, 45)
- High-volume suction/low-volume suction (p. 42, 43)
- Prophy handpiece (p. 74, 75)
- Bristle brush (p. 84) and rubber cup (p. 85)
- Flour of pumice to clean the tooth surface prior to sealant (do not use prophy paste as fluoride interferes with sealing procedure)
- Acid etch, sealant material
- Applicator brush (p. 90, 91)
- Glass dappen dish (p. 94, 95)
- Curing light (p. 108, 109)

SECTION 5

LOCAL ANAESTHESIA

Local anaesthetics provide temporary loss of sensation to a particular area of the mouth, so that the patient will not feel pain.

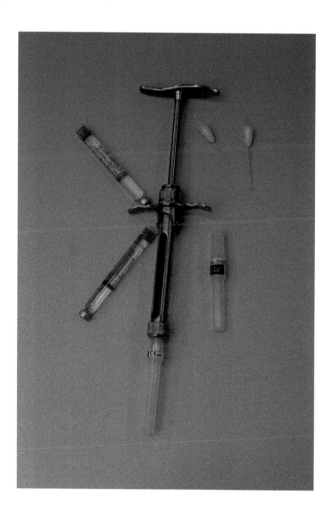

LOCAL ANAESTHESIA

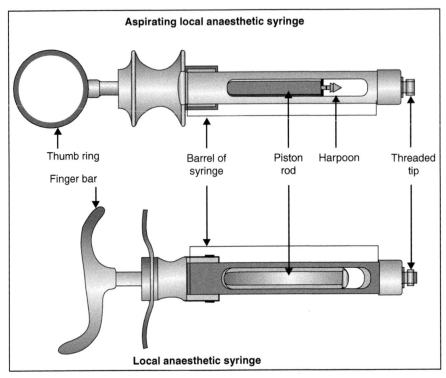

Figure 5.1

SYRINGES, NEEDLES AND CARTRIDGES

FIGURE 5.1

Name
Self-aspirating local anaesthetic syringe, Local anaesthetic syringe

Function and features
- A self-aspirating local anaesthetic syringe allows the operator to aspirate or draw back to see if they have injected into a blood vessel prior to injecting local anaesthetic, it is the harpoon or extension on the plunger which allows this. If the operator pulls towards themselves with the thumb ring, the 'draw back' action happens and if they depress the thumb ring it injects the local anaesthetic. If the operator 'draws back' and blood can be seen in the local anaesthetic carpule, they have injected into a blood vessel and will reposition prior to administering the local anaesthetic.
- Used to administer local anaesthetic with a disposable anaesthetic cartridge and a disposable needle
- The finger bar of the syringe controls the piston rod, which depresses the rubber stopper of the anaesthetic cartridge during aspiration
- When the piston rod is depressed, the local anaesthetic solution is forced out through the disposable needle, which is screwed onto the threaded tip
- The barrel of the syringe is open on both sides to facilitate loading the anaesthetic cartridge and check for blood cells during aspiration

Variations
Non-self-aspirating type, disposable type (assembled), top loading type, intraligamentary syringe

False friends
Irrigation syringe, endodontic syringe

LOCAL ANAESTHESIA

LOCAL ANAESTHESIA

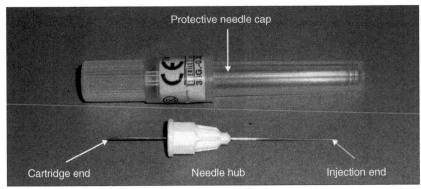

(a)

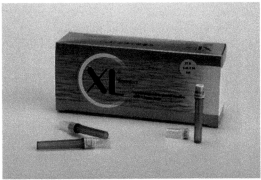

(b)

Figure 5.2

FIGURE 5.2a, b

Name
Disposable needle

Function, features and precautions
- Used in conjunction with a self-aspirating local anaesthetic syringe and disposable local anaesthetic cartridge
- Is threaded onto the hub of syringe – the short end of needle punctures the rubber diaphragm of the cartridge
- Single use
- Disposed of in the sharps' container
- Prior to use, check: seal is intact, expiry date and the length and gauge of the needle
- Lumen is the hollow centre of the needle
- Gauge is the thickness of the needle
- The type of injection dictates the appropriate length and gauge of needle to be used

Varieties
Available in different lengths and gauges

False friends
Irrigation syringe needle, endodontic syringe needle

LOCAL ANAESTHESIA

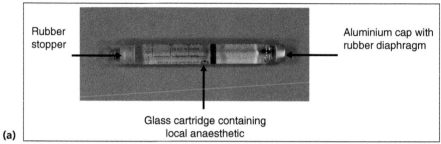

Rubber
stopper

Aluminium cap with
rubber diaphragm

Glass cartridge containing
local anaesthetic

(a)

LOCAL ANAESTHESIA

(b)

Figure 5.3

FIGURE 5.3a, b

Name
Glass disposable local anaesthetic cartridge

Function, precautions and contents
- Contains local anaesthetic solution for delivery
- Prior to use check: expiry date, cartridge and rubber diaphragm are intact and the clarity of the local anaesthetic solution (it should be clear)
- Single use
- Disposed in the sharps' container
- Contains water, preservatives, anaesthetic solution and buffering agents; some contain vasoconstrictors (Septodont products do not contain preservatives or latex)

Varieties
- Local anaesthetic constituents may vary

LOCAL ANAESTHESIA

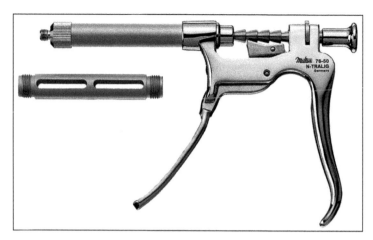

Figure 5.4

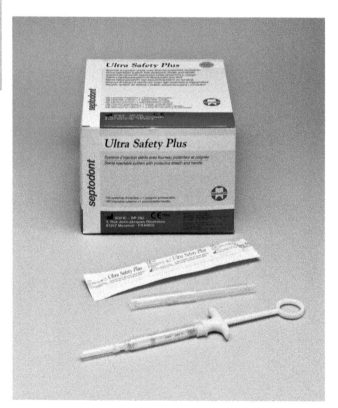

Figure 5.5

FIGURE 5.4

Name
Intraligamentary syringe

Functions and directions for use
- Used to deliver a small amount of local anaesthetic to a localised area
- A short or ultra-short needle is used with this syringe

Varieties
Different types of syringes available depending on the manufacturer

FIGURE 5.5

Name
Safety syringe

Functions and features
- Sterile, single-use syringe with an autoclavable handle
- A plastic sheath is used to cover the needle when not in use
- Designed to reduce the number of percutaneous injuries

Varieties
Different types of syringe available

LOCAL ANAESTHESIA

LOCAL ANAESTHESIA

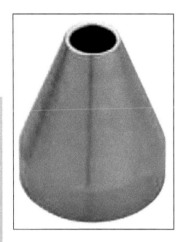

Figure 5.6

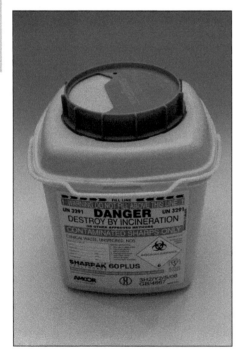

Figure 5.7

SHARPS' WASTE MANAGEMENT

FIGURE 5.6

Name
Needle stick protector

Function(s)
- A sturdy holder that holds the needle cap to facilitate safe recapping of the needle
- Designed to prevent percutaneous injuries
- A needle stick protector is not required if using the one-handed bayonet technique

Varieties
Many different types of needle stick protectors are available

FIGURE 5.7

Name
Sharps' disposal container

Functions, features and directions for use
- To safely dispose of sharps
- Must be puncture proof, closable, leak proof and colour coded
- Sharps' disposal containers should be placed close to work areas to prevent having to transport disposable sharp items
- Items suitable for disposal in these containers include scalpels, matrix bands, needles, carpules, orthodontic wires, burs and endodontic files

> **!** **Check your local health and safety guidelines for requirements of**
> **•** **sharps' disposal in your area**

LOCAL ANAESTHESIA

Set-up

Local anaesthetic

- Preferred type of local anaesthetic syringe
- Disposable local anaesthetic cartridge
- Disposable needle in desired length and gauge
- Needle holder (in case of needle breakage in the mouth) (p. 183, 184)
- Topical anaesthetic
- Topical anaesthetic applicator
- Disposable saliva ejector (p. 42, 43)

Optional: Special device for safe recapping of the disposable needle (only needed if not using the one-handed bayonet technique)

SECTION 6
INSTRUMENTS USED FOR RUBBER DAM PLACEMENT

A rubber dam is a thin sheet of material that is used to isolate the desired tooth or teeth to:
- aid moisture control
- protect the patient's airway
- aid operator visibility and access
- reduce aerosols caused by the air turbine handpiece
- provide patient comfort by reducing the amount of water and materials in the mouth

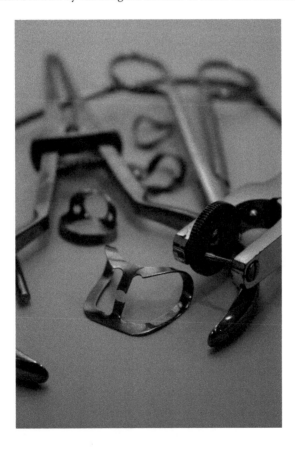

Basic Guide to Dental Instruments, Second Edition. Carmen Scheller-Sheridan.
© 2011 Carmen Scheller-Sheridan. Published 2011 by Blackwell Publishing Ltd.

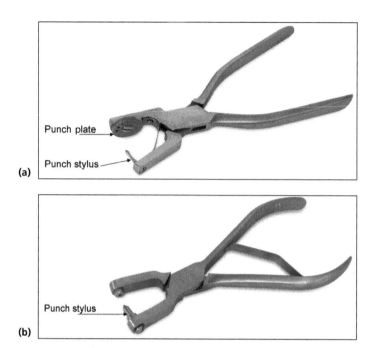

Figure 6.1

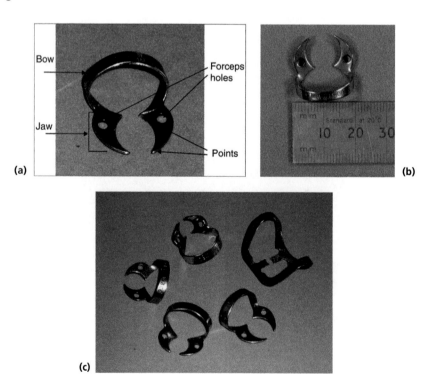

Figure 6.2

FIGURE 6.1a, b

Name
Rubber dam punch

Functions
- Used to perforate the rubber dam material with holes of various sizes corresponding to the size of the tooth to be isolated
- Size and position of the teeth to be isolated determines the orientation of the punched holes
- Punch stylus pierces a hole in the rubber dam sheet
- When the handle of the rubber dam punch is closed, the punch stylus meets the punch plate, which has serrated edges, to create a 'clean' punch

Varieties
- Available in various styles depending on the manufacturer
- In some styles, the punch stylus and plate can be replaced when they become dull (according to the manufacturer's specifications)

FIGURE 6.2a, b, c

Name
Rubber dam clamps

Functions and parts
- Used to stabilise and secure the rubber dam sheet during treatment
- Usually made from chrome- or nickel-plated steel – autoclavable
- Bow – rounds over the tooth. Varies between clamps and is flexible so that the clamp can have a firm hold on the tooth
- Jaw – the part of the rubber dam clamp that holds it firmly around the cervical portion of the tooth (pointed). Can be serrated for retention or smooth to prevent tissue trauma, and can be curved to fit sub-gingivally
- Forceps hole – where the rubber dam clamp forceps attach to the clamp for placement. Where a piece of floss can be tied to, in case of accidental displacement (the floss should be tied to both holes in case the bow breaks)

Varieties
- Various types, sizes and shapes (see figure for examples) available to use with teeth of different shapes
- Various degrees of flexibility

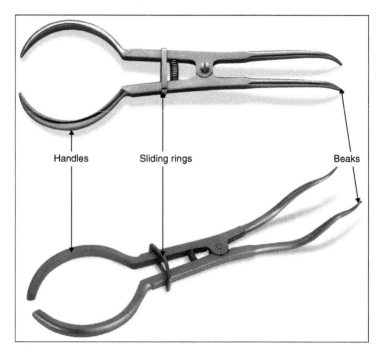

Handles   Sliding rings   Beaks

Figure 6.3

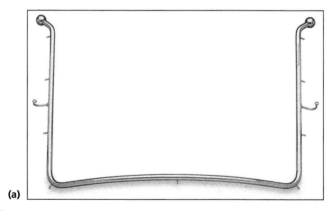

(a)

Figure 6.4

FIGURE 6.3

Name
Rubber dam clamp forceps

Functions and features
- Used to place and remove rubber dam clamps on and from a tooth
- Work with a spring action when handles are squeezed together
- Beaks – fit into the holes of the rubber dam clamp for secure placement
- Sliding ring – allows forceps to lock when placing the clamp and to be released when removing the clamp
- Handle – shaped to allow a firm palm-grasp by the operator

Varieties
- Available in various styles depending on the manufacturer

False friends
- Coon ligature pliers, separator placing pliers

FIGURE 6.4a, b

Name
Rubber dam frame: (a) Metal type (b) Plastic type

Function and feature
- Used to stretch the rubber dam to maintain a clear working area in the patient's mouth
- The rubber dam frame has extensions around which the rubber dam material is held

Varieties
- Available in various styles
- Can be made of different materials (e.g. metal and plastic)

INSTRUMENTS USED FOR RUBBER DAM PLACEMENT

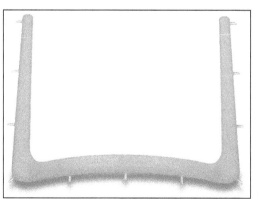

Figure 6.4 (*Continued*) **(b)**

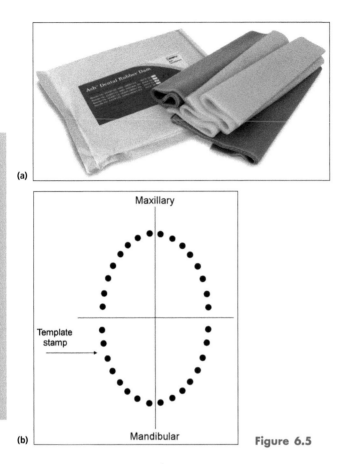

(a)

(b)

Figure 6.5

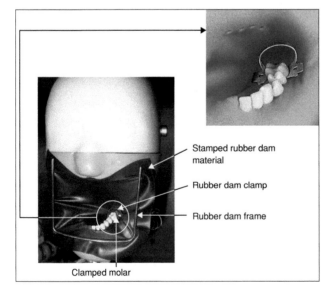

Figure 6.6

FIGURE 6.5a, b

Name
Rubber dam material (Figure 6.5a)

Functions and directions for use
- A thin sheet of latex or non-latex that aids with moisture control, infection control, airway protection, tissue and tongue retraction, patient comfort and operator visibility during treatment
- Is stretched around the rubber dam clamp seated in the mouth
- Can isolate one or many teeth depending on the procedure
- Waxed dental floss may be used to fit the septum of the rubber dam into the interproximal spaces of the tooth or teeth to be isolated
- May be stamped with a template (Figure 6.5b) to assist in punching the rubber dam

Varieties
- Various sizes and colours
- Various thicknesses
- Various materials

FIGURE 6.6

Mannequin with rubber dam in place

INSTRUMENTS USED FOR RUBBER
DAM PLACEMENT

Set-up

Set-up for placement of rubber dam
- Rubber dam material in desired thickness, stamping template
- Rubber dam punch
- Rubber dam clamp forceps
- Selected rubber dam clamps
- Rubber dam frame
- Blunt scissors/'Beebee' crown scissors/shears (p. 112, 113)
- Flat plastic instrument or another choice of blunt instrument (to help orientate rubber dam without puncturing) (p. 94, 95)
- Dental floss
- Gauze or napkins
- Lubricant (to aid in stretching the rubber dam material over the rubber dam clamp)
- Stabilising ligatures

SECTION 7

HANDPIECES, BURS AND ROTARY ATTACHMENTS

Dental handpieces and rotary attachments help to make dental treatment more comfortable for the patient and reduce the amount of time needed to complete procedures.

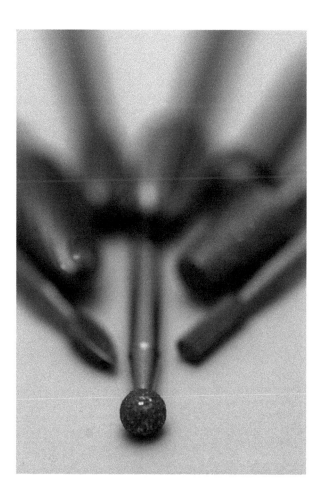

Basic Guide to Dental Instruments, Second Edition. Carmen Scheller-Sheridan.
© 2011 Carmen Scheller-Sheridan. Published 2011 by Blackwell Publishing Ltd.

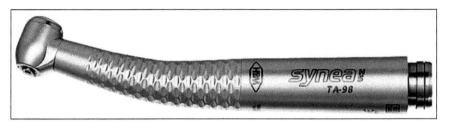

Figure 7.1

HANDPIECES

FIGURE 7.1

Name
Air turbine handpiece. Also called: fast handpiece, high-speed handpiece and air rotor handpiece

Type
Contra-angled

Functions, precaution and features
- Removal of tooth tissue during restorations and preparation of teeth for fixed prosthetic appliances
- Polishing of restorations
- High speeds create heat and friction – handpiece must be run with water to cool the tooth to prevent pulpal damage
- High speed saves treatment time and reduces vibration
- High speed but low torque handpiece will stall with moderate pressure

Driven by
- Turbine – may need to be lubricated – check manufacturer's instructions
- Compressed air rotates the turbine, which then rotates the bur

Speed
Check manufacturer's specifications (can run up to 500 000 rpm)

Grip
Accepts friction grip attachments

Attachment
Dental unit

Varieties
- Different types of chucks available (e.g. those which need bur changing tool)
- With or without light
- Smaller heads for difficult access or use with the paediatric patient

HANDPIECES, BURS AND
ROTARY ATTACHMENTS

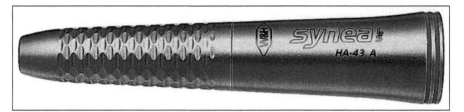

Figure 7.2

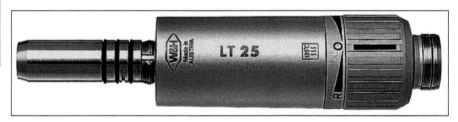

Figure 7.3

FIGURE 7.2

Name
Straight handpiece

Type
Straight

Functions
- Used in surgical procedures to remove bone (cannot use air turbine as the water is not sterile)
- Used extra-orally at chairside or in the dental laboratory (e.g. for denture adjustments)

Driven by
Gears

Speed
Check manufacturer's specifications (can run up to 40 000 rpm)

Grip
Accepts long shank attachments

Attachment
Electric motor that fits into the base of the handpiece

FIGURE 7.3

Name
Electric motor

Features
- Can reach speeds of 100 000 rpm depending on the type of attachment
- It is attached to the dental unit

HANDPIECES, BURS AND
ROTARY ATTACHMENTS

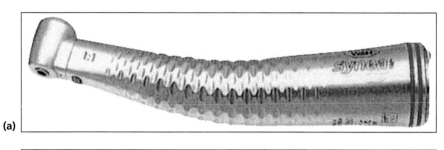

(a)

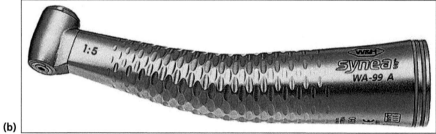

(b)

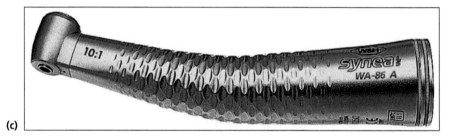

(c)

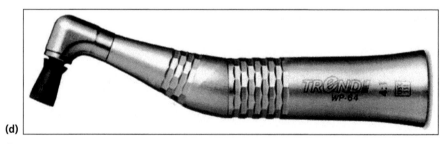

(d)

Figure 7.4

FIGURE 7.4a, b, c, d, e, f

Name
Conventional handpieces. Also called: slow-speed handpieces and low-speed handpieces

Type
Contra-angled

Functions
- Removal of caries
- Polishing
- Procedures that require torque
- Refine cavity preparations and adjust occlusion

Driven by
Gears

Speed
Varies depending on handpiece

Grip
Varies depending on handpiece

Attachment
Electric motor that fits into the base of the handpiece (see Figure 7.3)

Examples of conventional handpieces
Blue ring conventional handpiece (Figure 7.4a)
- Runs at the speed of the motor (up to 40 000 rpm)
- Accepts latch grip attachments
- Can have a latch chuck rather than a push type chuck

Orange ring conventional handpiece/variable speed handpiece (Figure 7.4b)
- Runs faster than the speed of the motor
- Accepts friction grip attachments

Green ring conventional handpiece/speed reducing handpiece (Figure 7.4c)
- Runs 10 times slower than the speed of the motor
- Accepts latch grip attachments

Prophy conventional handpiece (Figure 7.4d)
- Runs at the speed of the motor (40 000 rpm)
- Accepts screw type attachments
- Available with attachable, disposable prophy head (see pp. 266 and 267)

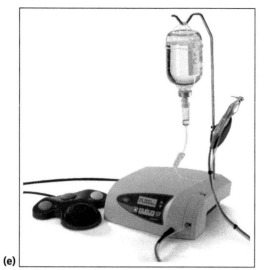

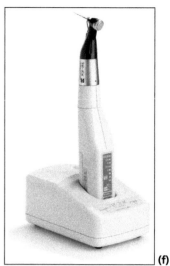

(e)

(f)

Figure 7.4 (*Continued*)

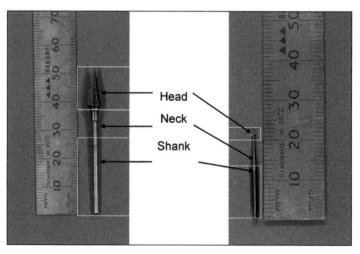

Head
Neck
Shank

Figure 7.5

Electric surgical and implant handpiece unit (Figure 7.4e)
- Runs at speeds of 40 000 rpm (varies with different handpieces)
- Can be used with straight and contra-angled handpieces for implant and maxillofacial surgery procedures
- Runs in conjunction with flowing sterile water during procedures

Endodontic handpiece (Figure 7.4f)
- Able to adjust the speed of the handpiece to run at very low speeds
- Used with specialised nickel–titanium rotary files to clean and shape root canals
- Handpiece in the illustration is a cordless handpiece with the motor in the unit, also available with separate unit

BURS AND ROTARY ATTACHMENTS

FIGURE 7.5

Enlarged view

Parts

Head
- This is the working end
- Function depends on the size and shape of the head
- Many different sizes and shapes, each used for a different function (cutting, polishing and finishing)

Neck
- The part that connects the head to the shank – usually narrows towards the head

Shank
- The part that fits into the handpiece
- Shapes and lengths vary, depending on function
- Can sometimes be marked to identify bur type (stripes or coloured bands)

Some points to remember about rotary attachments and burs
- Most often called burs, but also available are wheels, discs, rubber points, rubber cups and stones
- Each has a particular function (cutting, polishing, finishing or caries removal)
- Are made from various materials (tungsten carbide, diamond and steel)
- Can have flutes (the cutting edges)
- The end of the shank determines which handpiece the attachment will fit into:
  - Long straight shank – straight handpiece
  - Latch grip – conventional type/slow-speed handpiece
  - Friction grip shank – air turbine handpiece/high-speed handpiece
  - Other various attachments such as snap or screw-type attachments

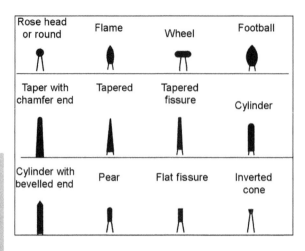

Rose head or round	Flame	Wheel	Football
Taper with chamfer end	Tapered	Tapered fissure	Cylinder
Cylinder with bevelled end	Pear	Flat fissure	Inverted cone

Figure 7.6

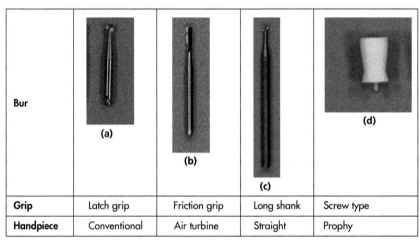

Bur	(a)	(b)	(c)	(d)
Grip	Latch grip	Friction grip	Long shank	Screw type
Handpiece	Conventional	Air turbine	Straight	Prophy

Figure 7.7

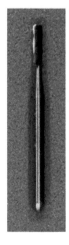

Figure 7.8

FIGURE 7.6

Some common shapes of dental burs

How to name and describe a dental bur
Five key characteristics:
(1) Grip of shank
(2) Composition of head
(3) Shape of head
(4) Function
(5) Handpiece that it fits

Grip and corresponding handpiece
Refers to the way the bur's shank is 'gripped' into the handpiece (Figure 7.7)

Composition
- Refers to the head of the bur and what it is made from
- Generally:
  - Most latch grip burs are made of steel
  - Most fiction grip burs are made of tungsten carbide or diamond
  - Most long shank burs are made from steel if they are meant for surgical procedures and stainless steel if they are meant for laboratory purposes

Shape and function
Shape determines function; the examples that follow relate to tungsten carbide burs:
- Rose head/round – cutting and removing caries
- Pear – to shape the cavity preparation
- Fissure – to shape and prepare the cavity preparation

Some examples follow.

FIGURE 7.8

Friction grip bur

Description
Friction grip, tungsten carbide, fissure, cutting bur for the air turbine handpiece

HANDPIECES, BURS AND ROTARY ATTACHMENTS

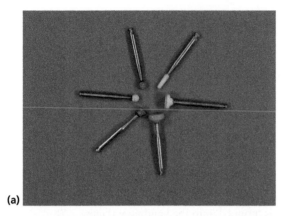

(a)

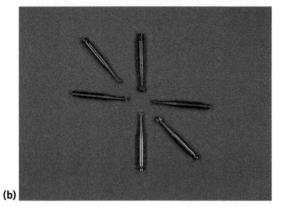

(b)   **Figure 7.9**

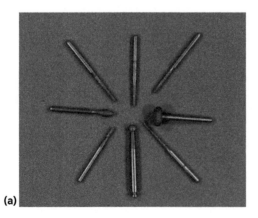

(a)   **Figure 7.10**

FIGURE 7.9a, b

Latch grip burs

Description
(a) Various shaped, latch grip, stone polishing burs for the conventional handpiece
(b) Various sizes of rose head/round, latch grip, steel cutting burs for the conventional handpiece

FIGURE 7.10a, b, c

Diamond burs

Description
Various shaped, friction grip, diamond cutting burs for the air turbine handpiece

HANDPIECES, BURS AND
ROTARY ATTACHMENTS

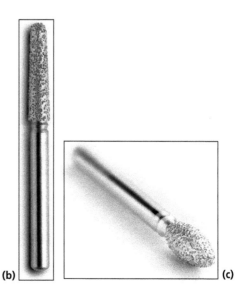

Figure 7.10 (*Continued*) **(b)** **(c)**

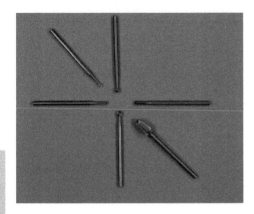

Figure 7.11

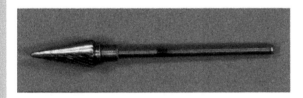

Figure 7.12

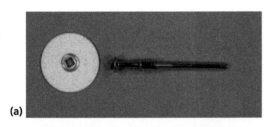

(a)

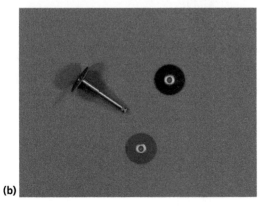

(b)   **Figure 7.13**

FIGURE 7.11

Long shank surgical burs

Description
Various shaped, long shank, steel cutting burs for the straight handpiece

FIGURE 7.12

Acrylic bur

Description
Used in laboratory procedures for cutting and trimming various materials. Available in many different shapes and sizes
- Illustration shows long shank, stainless steel, cone-shaped trimming bur for the straight handpiece

FIGURE 7.13a, b

Mandrels

Description
Discs for polishing and cutting are fitted onto mandrels. Discs can be either screw type (Moore mandrel and disc, Figure 7.13a) or pop-on type (mandrel and pop-on discs, Figure 7.13b)

HANDPIECES, BURS AND
ROTARY ATTACHMENTS

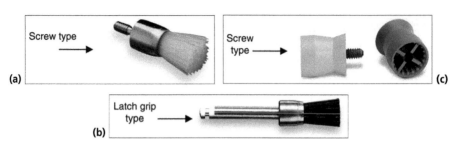

Figure 7.14

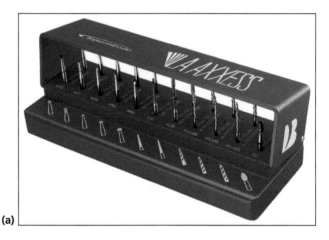

(a)

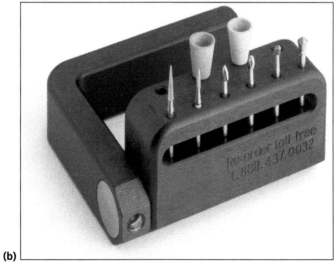

(b)

Figure 7.15

FIGURE 7.14a, b, c

Bristle brushes (Figure 7.14a, b), Rubber polishing cups (Figure 7.14c)

FIGURE 7.15a, b

Name
Bur blocks

Function and feature
- Used to organise and hold burs
- Some types are autoclavable

Varieties
- Different sizes and types available

HANDPIECES, BURS AND
ROTARY ATTACHMENTS

SECTION 8

INSTRUMENTS USED IN BASIC RESTORATIVE PROCEDURES

Basic restorative procedures involve placement of restorations where tooth tissue has been removed for a variety of reasons (e.g. fractures and caries)

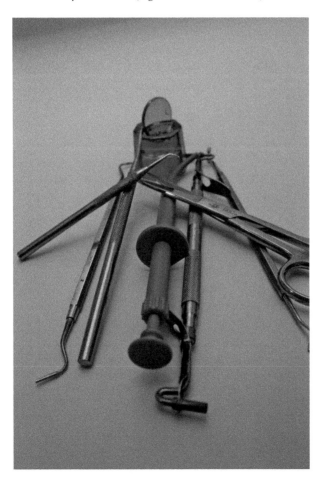

Basic Guide to Dental Instruments, Second Edition. Carmen Scheller-Sheridan.
© 2011 Carmen Scheller-Sheridan. Published 2011 by Blackwell Publishing Ltd.

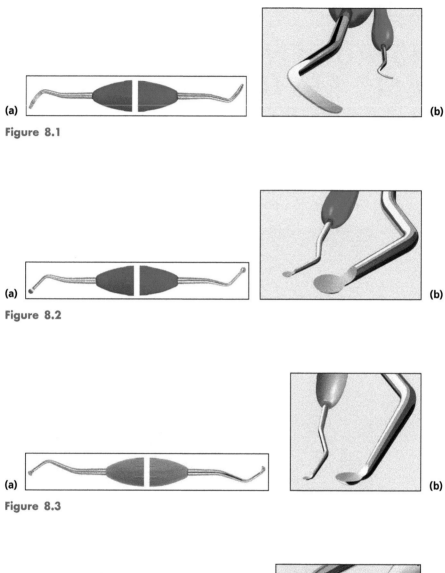

(a)   (b)

Figure 8.1

(a)   (b)

Figure 8.2

(a)   (b)

Figure 8.3

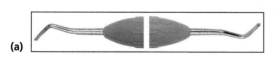
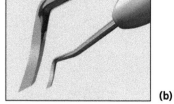

(a)   (b)

Figure 8.4

FOR ALL RESTORATIONS

FIGURES 8.1a, b; 8.2a, b; 8.3a, b

Name
Spoon excavators

Functions and feature
- A spoon-shaped working end for 'spooning' out dentinal caries from the cavity preparation
- Edges of working end are sharp

Any remaining caries will be removed with the conventional handpiece and a round bur

Varieties
Various sizes and shapes of working ends – can be double-ended or single-ended

False friends
Cleoid discoid carver, spoon curette, ball burnisher

FIGURES 8.4a, b; 8.5a, b

Name
Gingival margin trimmers (Figure 8.4a, b) Distal (Figure 8.5a, b) Mesial

Function and feature
- Used to remove unsupported enamel for refining the cavity preparation
- Sharp-bevelled working ends

False friends
Spoon excavator, Hollenback $3^1/_2$ carver, Wards carver

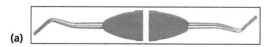

(a)

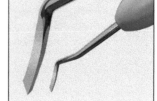

(b)

Figure 8.5

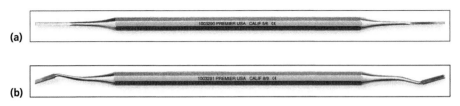

(a)

(b)

Figure 8.6

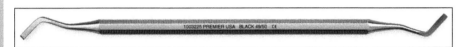

Figure 8.7

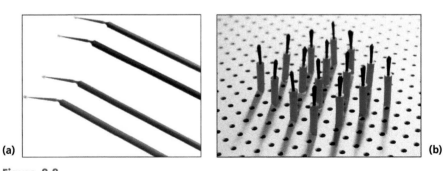

(a)   (b)

Figure 8.8

FIGURE 8.6a, b

Name
Enamel chisel

Function and feature
- Used to remove unsupported enamel for refining the cavity preparation
- Sharp-bevelled working ends

Varieties
Various sizes and shapes available

False friends
Push scaler, ligature tucker

FIGURE 8.7

Name
Enamel hatchet

Function and feature
- Used to remove unsupported enamel for refining the cavity preparation
- Working end is on the same plane as the handle

Varieties
Various sizes and shapes available

False friends
Push scaler, gingival margin trimmer, enamel chisel

FIGURE 8.8a, b

Name
Disposable applicators

Function(s)
- Used to apply materials intra-orally, e.g. desensitising agents, bonding agents and cavity varnish
- 8.8b are inserted into a plastic handle

Varieties
Many different types and shapes available

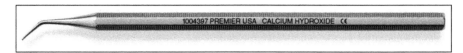

Figure 8.9

(a)

(b)

(c)

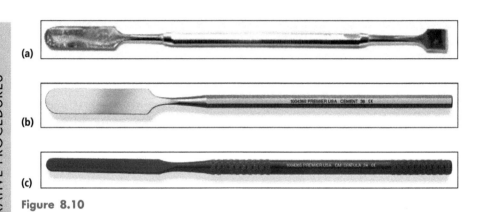

Figure 8.10

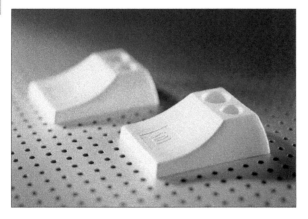

Figure 8.11

FIGURE 8.9

Name
Calcium hydroxide applicator

Function
• Used to apply calcium hydroxide and other lining materials at the base of the cavity preparation

Varieties
Different sized working ends and long handles available

FIGURE 8.10a, b, c

Name
Mixing spatulas: (a) Stainless steel Weston spatula (b) Stainless steel broad bladed spatula (c) Anodised aluminium spatula

Function and feature
• Used to mix dental materials
• Anodised aluminium spatula will not stick to any composite materials or discolour materials (Figure 8.10c)

Varieties
Different sizes, degrees of flexibility and shapes available

FIGURE 8.11

Name
Dispensing wells

Function
• Used to hold material to be dispensed (e.g. bonding agent)

Varieties
• Available in various shapes and sizes
• Available with a small orange shield over dispensing hole to protect dispensed materials from light
• Available as disposable type

INSTRUMENTS USED IN BASIC RESTORATIVE PROCEDURES

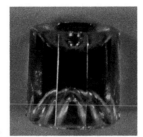

(a)

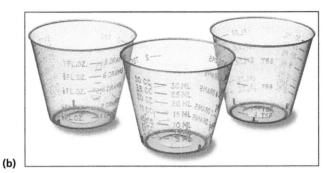

(b)

Figure 8.12

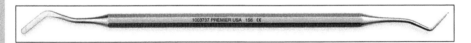

Figure 8.13

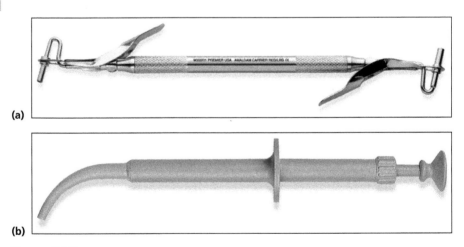

(a)

(b)

Figure 8.14

FIGURE 8.12a, b

Name
(a) Glass dappen dish (b) Disposable plastic dappen dishes

Function
To hold materials for dispensing

Varieties
Various shapes, sizes and colours available

FOR AMALGAM RESTORATIONS

FIGURE 8.13

Name
Flat plastic instrument. Also called: plastic instrument

Functions
- To deliver materials to the cavity preparation
- To remove excess materials

Varieties
- Various sizes and shapes available
- Can be single-ended or double-ended

False friends
Spoon excavator, Hollenback $3\frac{1}{2}$ carver, Wards carver

FIGURE 8.14a, b

Name
(a) Metal amalgam carrier (b) Plastic amalgam carrier

Function, features and precaution
- Used to pick up, transport and place amalgam into the cavity preparation
- Working end is hollow
- A plunger/lever pushes amalgam out from working end into the cavity preparation
- The working end may be Teflon$^{\circledR}$ coated so the amalgam will not stick
- Care must be taken to expel the excess amalgam or it will set inside the working end
- Sterilisation procedures may vary depending on the material that the amalgam carrier is fabricated from

Varieties
- Various delivery methods
- Various sizes of working ends for different amounts of amalgam needed
- Can be single-ended or double-ended

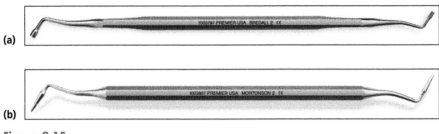

(a)

(b)

Figure 8.15

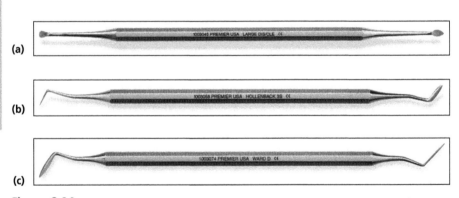

(a)

(b)

(c)

Figure 8.16

FIGURE 8.15a, b

Name
(a) Universal Hobsons plugger (b) Mortonson-Clevedent plugger

Family
Amalgam pluggers/condensers

Function and feature
- To pack and condense amalgam into a cavity preparation
- Working ends are flat
- The size and shape of the cavity preparation will dictate which plugger is required

Varieties
- Various sizes and working ends
- Can be single-ended or double-ended

FIGURE 8.16a, b, c

Name
(a) Cleoid Discoid carver (b) Hollenback $3^1/_2$ carver (c) Wards carver

Family
Carvers

Function and feature
- Used to carve and shape the amalgam restoration for correct anatomy and occlusion
- Edges of working ends are sharp
- Operator preference and shape of restoration will dictate which carver is required

Varieties
- Various sizes and working ends
- Can be single-ended or double-ended

INSTRUMENTS USED IN BASIC RESTORATIVE PROCEDURES

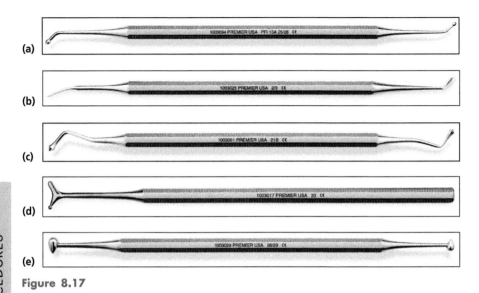

(a)

(b)

(c)

(d)

(e)

Figure 8.17

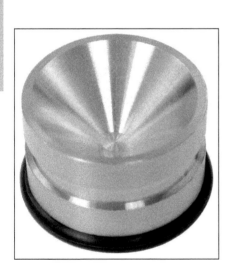

Figure 8.18

FIGURE 8.17a, b, c, d, e

Name
(a) Ball burnisher (b) Beavertail burnisher (c) Acorn burnisher (d) T-ball burnisher (e) Egg ball/football burnisher

Family
Burnishers

Function and feature
- Polish and smooth amalgam once condensed in prepared cavity
- Adapt amalgam to the margins of restorations, reducing the chance for leakage around restorations and deficient margins
- The working end is smooth and rounded

Varieties
- Various sizes of working ends
- Can be single-ended or double-ended

False friend
Spoon excavator

FIGURE 8.18

Name
Amalgam well

Function(s)
- Used to hold amalgam and to facilitate filling of the amalgam carrier

Varieties
- Various shapes
- Available in plastic, disposable variety

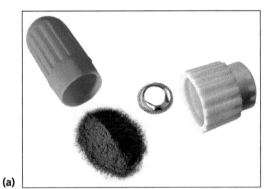

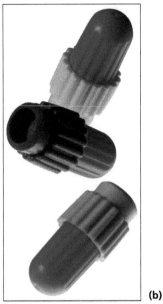

(a)

(b)

Figure 8.19

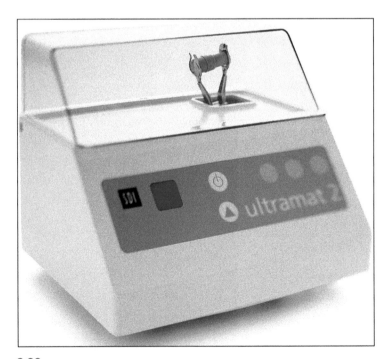

Figure 8.20

FIGURES 8.19a, b; 8.20

Name
Amalgam capsule (Figure 8.19a, b) Amalgamator (Figure 8.20)

Functions and precautions
- An amalgam capsule contains amalgam material (contents will vary depending on the manufacturer)
- Care must be taken when handling amalgam to prevent inhalation of vapours, skin absorption and inhalation of air-borne particles
- Amalgamator is used to titrate amalgam prior to use
- Amalgamators must have a plastic covering over the area where the amalgam is titrated for safety in case of displacement

Varieties
- Available in different delivery systems
- Different spills (amount of amalgam contained), i.e. 1 spill and 2 spills available
- Amalgamators vary depending on manufacturer

AMALGAM WASTE MANAGEMENT

FIGURE 8.21

Name
Amalgam Safe® container

Function
Airtight containers with foam inserts that contain non-hazardous chemicals that will suppress mercury vapours

Varieties
Other different types available depending on the manufacturer

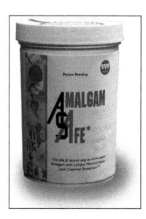

Figure 8.21

INSTRUMENTS USED IN BASIC
RESTORATIVE PROCEDURES

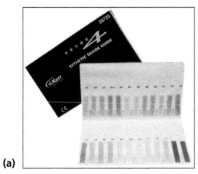
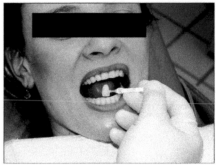

(a)   (b)

Figure 8.22

INSTRUMENTS USED IN BASIC
RESTORATIVE PROCEDURES

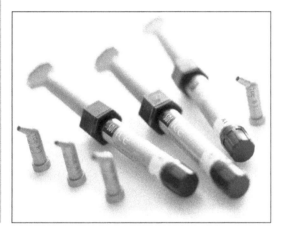

Figure 8.23

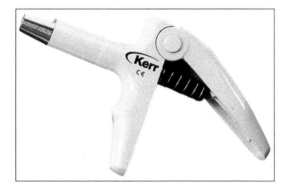

Figure 8.24

FOR COMPOSITE RESTORATIONS

FIGURE 8.22a, b

Name
(a) Shade guide (b) Checking the shade of a patient's tooth

Functions, feature and directions for use
- Used to match the colour of the patient's natural tooth
- The tabs are coded with numbers or a combination of numbers and letters, e.g. shade A3
- The shade is then recorded on the laboratory slip chart and patient chart so the lab technician can match the colour of the prosthesis (e.g. crown or denture) or restoration to the shade of the patient's natural tooth

Varieties
Different manufacturers have different varieties of shade guides for their own products

FIGURE 8.23

Name
Composite material

Function, feature and precaution
- Available as unidose capsules or bulk tubes
- Capsules are designed for easy delivery of composite material to the cavity preparation with a composite gun
- Composite capsules are for single use
- Only sterile instruments should be used when dispensing composite from a bulk tube to prevent contamination of material

Varieties
Various brands and shades available

FIGURE 8.24

Name
Composite gun

Function and precaution
- For easy delivery of composite material
- Used in conjunction with unidose composite capsules
- Care must be taken when autoclaving (follow manufacturer's instructions)

Varieties
Various shapes available

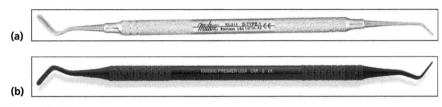

Figure 8.25

INSTRUMENTS USED IN BASIC
RESTORATIVE PROCEDURES

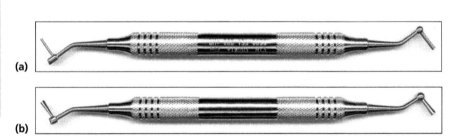

Figure 8.26

FIGURE 8.25a, b

Name
Composite flat plastic: (a) Teflon type (b) Anodised aluminium type. Also called: plastic instrument

Functions
- Available as anodised aluminium or Teflon coated. These are suitable for use with composite as they do not stick to or discolour composite material
- To deliver materials to the cavity preparation
- To adapt filling materials to a cavity preparation
- To remove excess materials

Varieties
- Various sizes and shapes are available
- Can be single-ended or double-ended

False friends
Spoon excavator, Hollenback $3\frac{1}{2}$ carver, Wards carver

FIGURE 8.26a, b

Name
Teflon-tipped super pluggers

Family
Composite pluggers/condensers

Function and features
- To pack and condense composite into a cavity preparation
- Working ends are flat, with a burnisher-type end on the angle of the shank
- Teflon coated so they will not stick to or discolour composite material

Varieties
- Various sizes and working ends available
- Can be single ended or double ended

INSTRUMENTS USED IN BASIC RESTORATIVE PROCEDURES

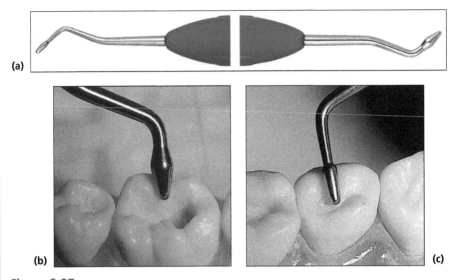

Figure 8.27

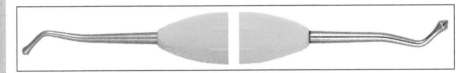

Figure 8.28

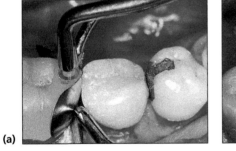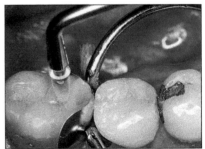

Figure 8.29

FIGURES 8.27a, b, c; 8.28

Name
Modelling instrument (Figure 8.27a, b, c) Acorn burnisher (Figure 8.28)

Functions and feature
- Used to create anatomical shapes in composite material during restorations
- The modelling instrument can also be used to pack and condense composite materials
- Available in plastic autoclavable type through which the curing light can penetrate

Varieties
- Various sizes and shapes of working ends available
- Can be single-ended or double-ended

FIGURE 8.29a, b

Name
Contact former

Function and precaution while in use
- Used to help create a good interproximal contact between adjacent teeth
- After the initial placement of composite, the instrument is placed in the composite in the desired location. The composite is then light cured, care must be taken to place the instrument in such a way that it will not get stuck in the composite

Varieties
- Available as plastic autoclavable type through which the curing light can penetrate
- Various sizes and shapes of working ends available
- Can be single-ended or double-ended

False friends
Acorn burnisher, Acorn carver

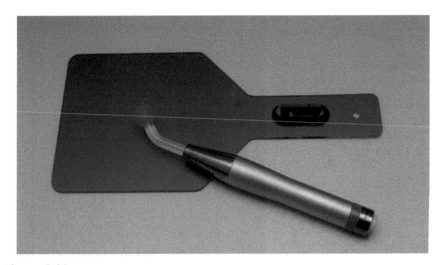

Figure 8.30

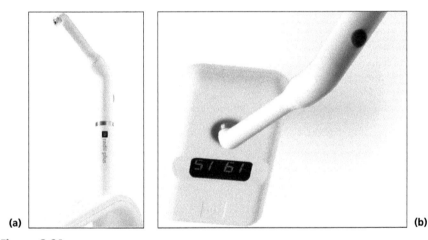

(a)   (b)

Figure 8.31

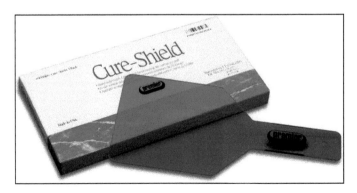

Figure 8.32

FIGURE 8.30

Name
Halogen curing light

Function and precautions
- Used to harden (cure) certain materials (e.g. composite, bonding agents, sealants and core build-ups)
- Materials should be built up and cured in increments of 2 mm
- Curing light can be monitored for safe and efficient operating
- Must be used with amber shield for eye protection

Varieties
Different manufacturers supply different types of halogen curing light

FIGURE 8.31a, b

Name
(a) LED (light-emitting diode) curing light (b) Radiometer

Functions, features and precaution
- Used to harden certain materials (e.g. composite, bonding agents, sealants and core build-ups)
- Generate light in wavelengths
- Curing light can be monitored for safe and efficient operating using a radiometer
- Cures at a high density allowing a greater depth of curing
- Must be used with amber shield for eye protection

Varieties
Different manufacturers supply different types of LED curing light (the illustrated light is cordless)

FIGURE 8.32

Name
Amber shield

Functions
- Used to protect eyes from the curing light
- The orange colour blocks the harmful light

Varieties
Available as safety glasses

INSTRUMENTS USED IN BASIC RESTORATIVE PROCEDURES

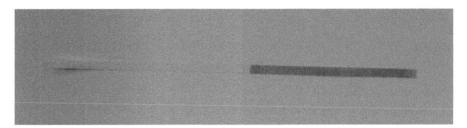

Figure 8.33

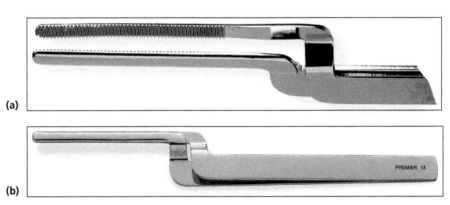

(a)

(b)

Figure 8.34

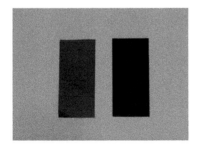

Figure 8.35

FIGURE 8.33

Name
Composite polishing/finishing strip

Function and features
- To smooth and polish composite interproximally after final curing
- One strip has varying degrees of abrasiveness
- Single use
- Can also be used in conjunction with periodontal treatment to remove stain interproximally where there is a tight contact

Varieties
Various widths and abrasiveness available

FOR ALL RESTORATIONS AGAIN

FIGURE 8.34a, b

Name
(a) Miller's articulating forceps (working end) (b) Miller's articulating forceps in closed position

Function and precaution
- To secure the articulating paper in place while checking the occlusion
- The articulating paper should be 5 mm longer than the Miller forceps, if checking occlusion on posterior teeth. This is due to the patient closing down and causing discomfort by hitting off the end of the Miller's forceps, if the articulating paper is not extended

False friend
College tweezers

FIGURE 8.35

Name
Articulating paper

Function
Carbon paper used to create a mark on a surface of a restoration or prosthesis that is interfering with the correct occlusion of the maxillary and mandibular teeth

Varieties
- Various colours and thicknesses available
- Available pre-cut or in a roll

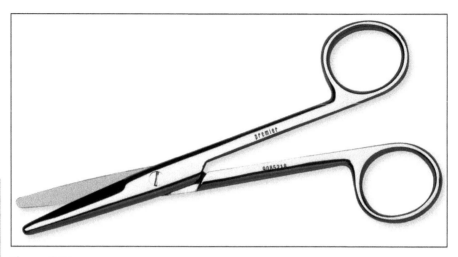

Figure 8.36

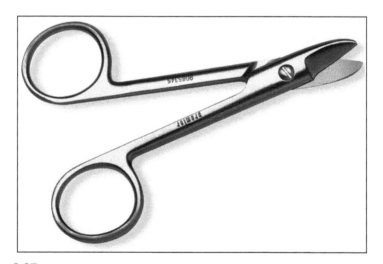

Figure 8.37

FIGURE 8.36

Name
Straight blunt scissors

Function and feature
- Cutting
- One side of blade is blunt and one is pointed to prevent causing trauma to the patient

Varieties
Different shapes and sizes available

False friend
Surgical scissors

FIGURE 8.37

Name
Beebee crown scissors/shears

Function
Cutting and trimming various materials, e.g. rubber dam septa, provisional/temporary crowns

Varieties
Various shapes and sizes available

Set-ups

The following instruments are common to all the below listed set-ups:
- Mouth mirror and handle (p. 34, 35)
- Sickle/contra-angled probe (p. 36, 37)
- College tweezers (p. 39, 40)
- High and low volume/disposable saliva ejector suction tips (p. 42, 43)
- Instruments for local anaesthetic set-up (see Section 5, p. 49)
- Instruments for rubber dam set-up (see Section 6, p. 61)
- Spoon excavator
- Enamel chisels and gingival margin trimmers
- Air turbine handpiece (p. 70, 71)
- Conventional handpiece (p. 74, 75)
- Various burs (see Section 7, p. 69)
- Various base and liner materials
- Flat plastic instrument
- Air/water syringe/3-in-1 syringe (p. 46, 47)
- Wooden wedges/plastic wedges (p. 120, 121)
- Miller forceps and articulating paper
- Dental floss

Amalgam restoration
- Amalgam carrier
- Amalgam pluggers
- Amalgam carvers
- Amalgam burnishers
- Matrix retainer and appropriate matrix material (see Section 9, p. 115)
- Amalgam well/glass dappen dish

Composite restoration
- Shade guide
- Teflon tipped flat plastic instrument
- Celluloid strip/clear transparent matrix strip (see Section 9, p. 116, 117)
- Composite polishing/finishing strip
- Mandrel and pop-on sandpaper discs
- Light-curing unit
- Amber shield
- Composite polishing and finishing burs (see Section 7, p. 69)

Posterior composites
- Clear proximal matrices (see Section 9, p. 116, 117)
- Light-reflecting wedges (p. 120, 121)
- Sectional matrices and BiTineTM rings (see Section 9, p. 124, 125)
- Contact formers

SECTION 9
MATRIX BANDS AND MATRIX RETAINERS

When a restoration involves an interproximal surface, it is not possible to achieve a properly adapted restoration without a matrix band. A matrix band creates a temporary interproximal surface, and, when appropriate, a matrix retainer secures the matrix band in place.

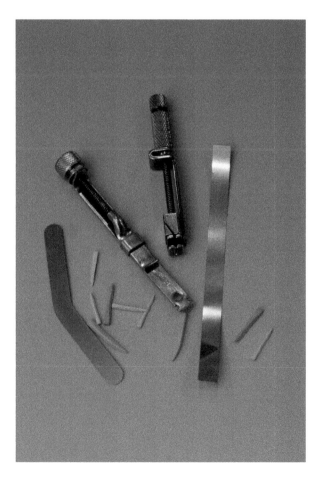

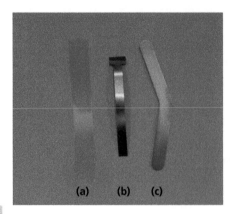

Figure 9.1

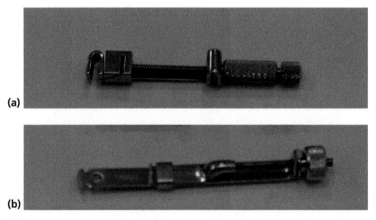

Figure 9.2

FIGURE 9.1a, b, c

Name
Matrix material

Function
Used to form a temporary wall where a proximal surface has been removed or is missing

Varieties
(a) Celluloid strip
  - Used for anterior restorations with composite materials
  - Also referred to as clear transparent matrix strip
  - Single use
  - Disposed of in the sharps' container
  - Preformed posterior variety can be available (see Sectional matrix, Figure 9.3)
(b) T-band matrix (straight and curved)
  - Most commonly used in paedodontics
  - Single use
  - Disposed of in the sharps' container
(c) Stainless steel matrix band (universal)
  - Used in conjunction with amalgam restorations and a matrix retainer
  - Single use
  - Disposed of in the sharps' container
  - Different sizes and shapes available
  - Available in pre-contoured shapes

FIGURE 9.2a, b

Name
(a) Tofflemire matrix retainer (b) Siqveland matrix retainer

Function and features
- Used to hold a stainless steel matrix band securely
- Assembled to fit in a particular quadrant of the mouth
- Autoclavable

Varieties
Can be available in disposable plastic

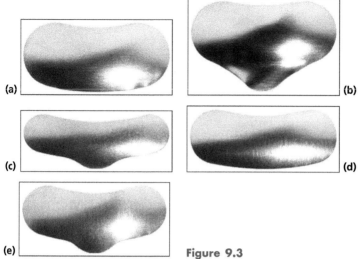

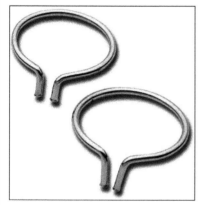

(a) (b) (c) (d) (e)

Figure 9.3

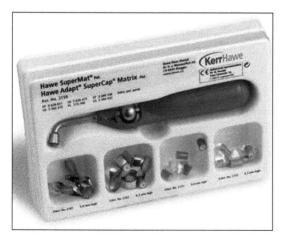

Figure 9.4

Figure 9.5

FIGURES 9.3a, b, c, d, e; 9.4

Name
Sectional matrix (Figures 9.3a, b, c, d, e) and BiTine™ ring (Figure 9.4)

Function and features
- Used in conjunction with posterior restorations to temporarily replace proximal walls during Class II restorations
- Available in four sizes: paedodontic, bicuspids, smaller molars and standard molars
- The matrices are shaped to conform to tooth shape

Varieties
Many different systems available

FIGURE 9.5

Name
Hawe Supermat Matrix®

Function and features
- Used in conjunction with posterior composite and amalgam restorations to temporarily replace proximal walls during restorations
- Available in different sizes to adapt to different sized teeth
- Available in stainless steel and clear matrix materials
- The matrices are shaped to conform to tooth shape

Varieties
Many other different types available from different manufacturers

MATRIX BANDS AND MATRIX RETAINERS

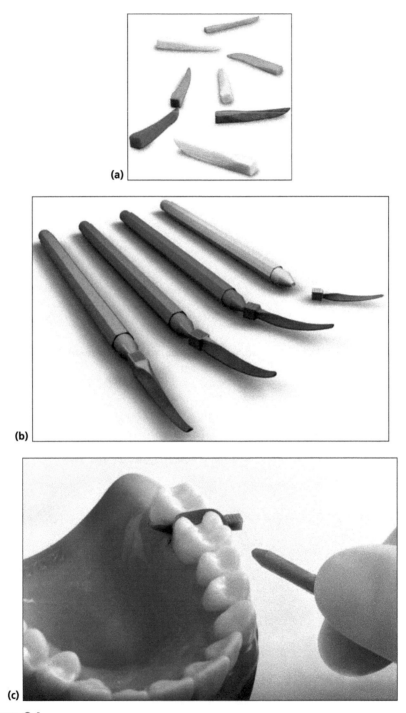

Figure 9.6

FIGURE 9.6a, b, c

Name
(a) Wooden wedges (b) Plastic wedges

Functions and features
- Used in conjunction with a matrix band, sectional matrix or celluloid strip
- Help to support and adapt the matrix to the tooth
- Assist in maintaining adequate contact points between two adjacent teeth
- Essential for the elimination of overhangs
- Single use
- Disposed of in the sharps' container

Varieties
Various sizes, shapes and materials

FIGURE 9.7

Name
Light-reflecting wedges

Functions and features
- Used in conjunction with a matrix band and composite restorations
- Reflect the light from the curing light onto the composite material
- Help support and adapt the matrix to the tooth
- Assist in maintaining adequate contact points between two adjacent teeth
- Essential for the elimination of overhangs
- Single use
- Disposed of in the sharps' container

Varieties
Various sizes and shapes available

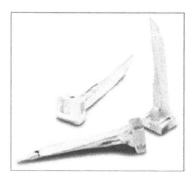

Figure 9.7

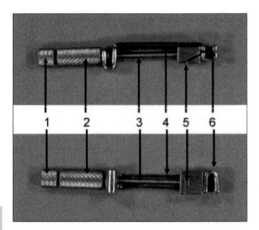

Figure 9.8

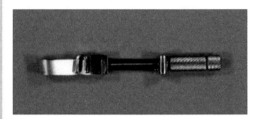

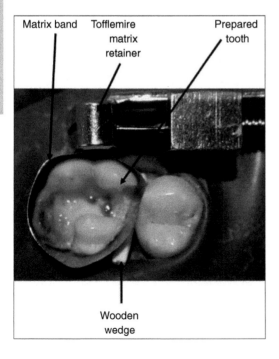

Figure 9.9

Figure 9.10

TOFFLEMIRE MATRIX RETAINER AND STAINLESS STEEL MATRIX BAND SET-UP

FIGURE 9.8

Parts of a Tofflemire matrix retainer

(1) Outer nut – Used to tighten or loosen the spindle to hold the matrix band
(2) Inner nut – Used to change the size of the matrix band by adjusting the position to fit a specific tooth
(3) Spindle – A straight screw used to secure the matrix band
(4) Frame – Hold the parts of the matrix retainer together
(5) Guide slot – Diagonal slot where the matrix band is placed and is secured by the spindle
(6) Outer guide slots – Extensions that aid in the positioning of the matrix band in left, right or anterior/universal positions

FIGURE 9.9

Tofflemire matrix retainer with matrix band in the universal position

FIGURE 9.10

Tooth with Tofflemire retainer and matrix band in place

FIGURE 9.11a, b

Name

(a) Celluloid strip in place (b) Light curing an anterior restoration through a celluloid strip

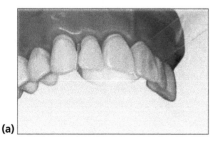
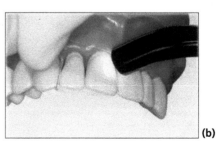

(a)   (b)

Figure 9.11

MATRIX BANDS AND MATRIX RETAINERS

MATRIX BANDS AND MATRIX RETAINERS

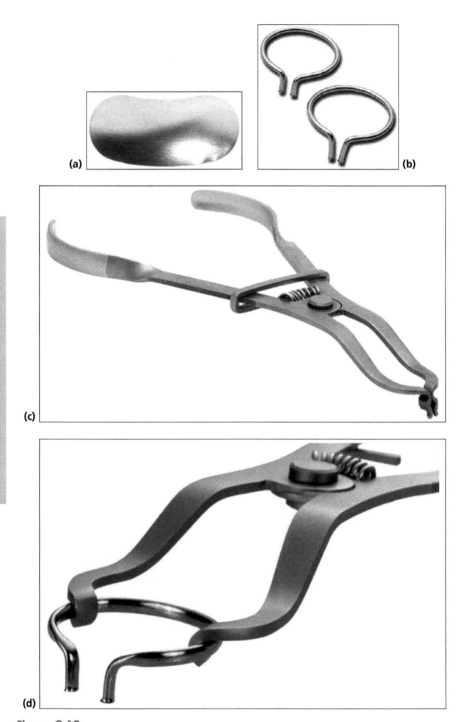

(a)

(b)

(c)

(d)

Figure 9.12

SECTIONAL MATRIX AND BITINE RING SET-UP

FIGURE 9.12a, b, c, d

Sectional matrix and BiTine ring set-up

Consists of
- Sectional matrix (Figure 9.3a)
- BiTine ring (Figure 9.3b)
- Special ring placement instrument

FIGURE 9.13

Tooth with sectional matrix, plastic wedges and BiTine rings in place

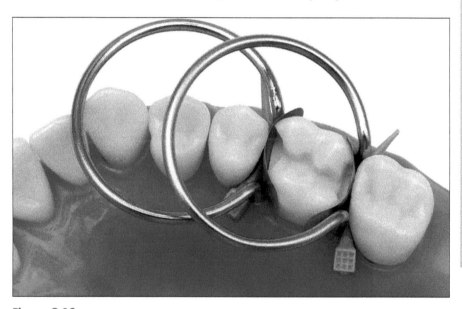

Figure 9.13

MATRIX BANDS AND MATRIX RETAINERS

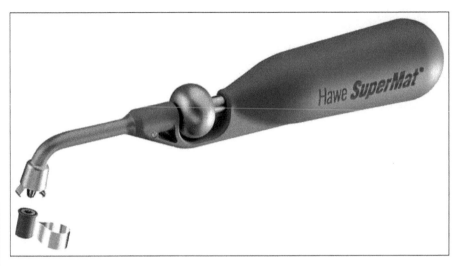

Figure 9.14

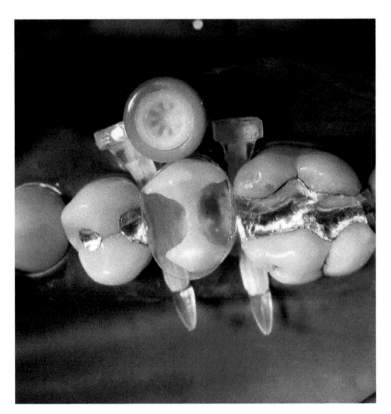

Figure 9.15

HAWE SUPERMAT MATRIX SET-UP

FIGURE 9.14

Hawe Supermat Matrix set-up

Consists of
- Pre-formed matrix bands of various shapes in both stainless steel and clear matrix
- Special tool to tighten and release matrix band (Figure 9.14)

FIGURE 9.15

Hawe Supermat Matrix and light reflecting wedges in place

MATRIX BANDS AND MATRIX RETAINERS

Set-up

Set-up for using matrix retainers and matrix bands (in conjunction with a restoration set-up)

- Mouth mirror and handle (p. 34, 35)
- Sickle/contra-angled probe (p. 36, 37)
- College tweezers (p. 39, 40)
- Matrix band – select the appropriate type
- Matrix retainer – if necessary
- Burnisher – to burnish the band if it has been bent (p. 98, 99)
- Wooden, plastic or light-reflecting wedges – select proper size and shape
- Beebee crown scissors/shears (p. 112, 113)

SECTION 10

INSTRUMENTS USED IN ENDODONTIC TREATMENT

When the pulp suffers irreversible pulpitis, the only way to retain the natural tooth is by complete removal of the pulp.

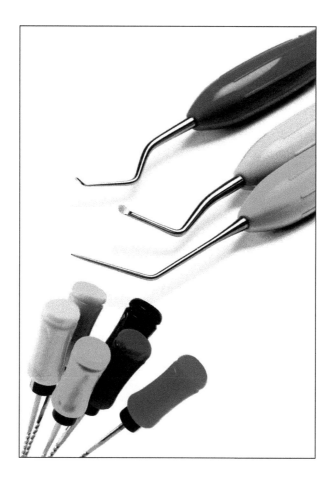

Basic Guide to Dental Instruments, Second Edition. Carmen Scheller-Sheridan.
© 2011 Carmen Scheller-Sheridan. Published 2011 by Blackwell Publishing Ltd.

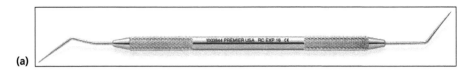

(a)

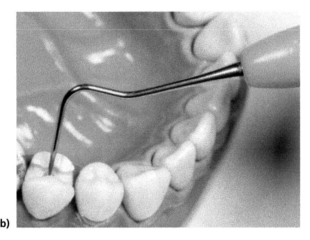

(b)

Figure 10.1

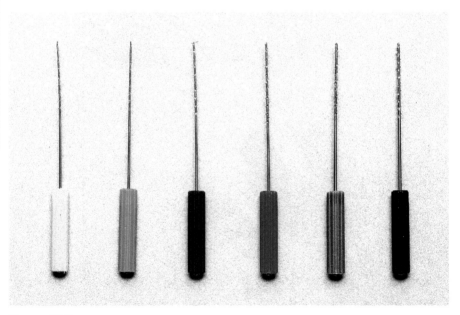

Figure 10.2

ENDODONTIC INSTRUMENTS

FIGURE 10.1a, b

Name
DG16 probe/root canal explorer

Function
Used to probe and detect canal openings within the pulp chamber

False friends
Root canal spreader, sickle/contra-angled probe

FIGURE 10.2

Name
Barbed broaches

Functions and precautions
- Single use finger instruments
- Disposed of in the sharps' container
- Used to remove the intact pulp
- 'Barbs' on the broach snag the pulp to facilitate removal
- They need to be used cautiously as they can bind and break in the canal

Varieties
Available in different sizes and widths

False friends
Endodontic K files, Hedström files (used as an alternative), finger spreaders

INSTRUMENTS USED IN ENDODONTIC TREATMENT

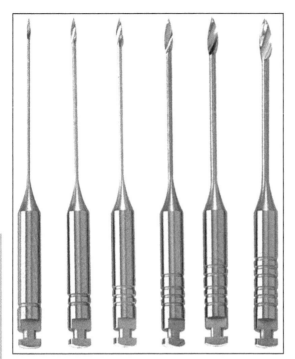

Figure 10.3

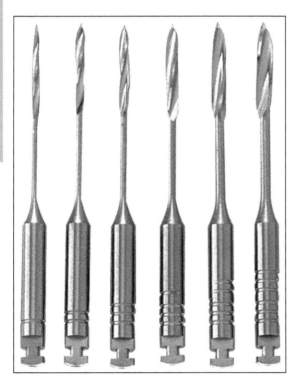

Figure 10.4

FIGURE 10.3

Name
Gates Glidden drills

Function, features and precautions
- To enlarge the coronal third of the canal during endodontic treatment
- Small flame-shaped cutting instrument used in the conventional handpiece
- Different sizes – coded by rings or coloured bands on shank
- Are slightly flexible and will follow the canal shape but can perforate the canal if used too deeply
- Dispose of in sharps' container and are single use
- Should be used only in the straight sections of the canal

False friend
Peeso reamer drill

FIGURE 10.4

Name
Peeso reamer drills

Function, features and precautions
- To remove gutta percha during post-preparation
- Small flame-shaped cutting instrument used in the conventional handpiece
- Different sizes – coded by rings or coloured bands on shank
- Peeso reamers are not flexible or adaptable, if not used with care can perforate canal
- Dispose of in sharps' container

False friend
Gates Glidden drill

INSTRUMENTS USED IN
ENDODONTIC TREATMENT

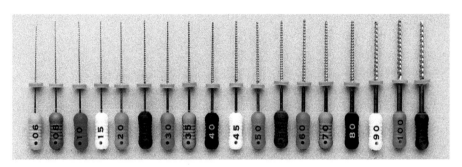

Figure 10.5

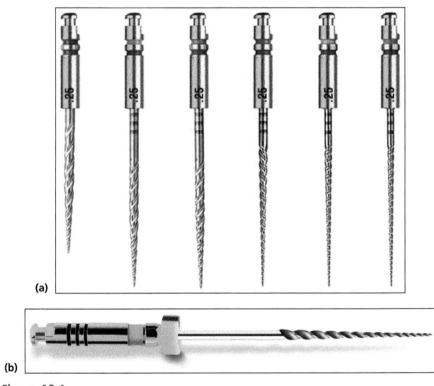

(a)

(b)

Figure 10.6

FIGURE 10.5

Name
Endodontic K files. Also called: root canal hand files

Function, features and precaution
- Finger instrument
- Colour coded by size. The six colours used most often are: size 15 (white), 20 (yellow), 25 (red), 30 (blue), 35 (green) and 40 (black). Also available in size 6 (pink), 8 (grey) and 10 (purple)
- Operator gradually increases the size of the file to smooth, shape and enlarge canal
- The larger the number of the file, the larger the diameter of the working end
- Disposed of in the sharps' container and are single use

Varieties
- Different lengths: 21 mm, 25 mm and 30 mm
- Hedström files, Flexofiles®

False friends
Barbed broaches, finger spreaders

FIGURE 10.6a, b

Name
NiTi (Nickel titanium) rotary instruments

Function, features and directions for use
- Used to clean and shape the canals
- Used with endodontic handpiece and motor (see Section 7)
- NiTi is flexible and instruments follow the canal outline very well
- Several varieties of systems with different sequences of instruments are used
- Important to follow the manufacturer's recommended speeds and instructions for use

Varieties
Different lengths: 21 mm and 25 mm

False friends
Gates Glidden drills, Peeso reamer drills

INSTRUMENTS USED IN
ENDODONTIC TREATMENT

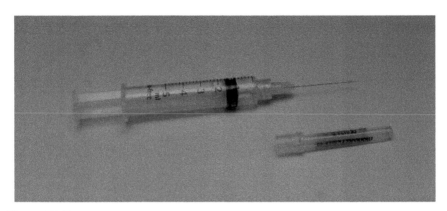

Figure 10.7

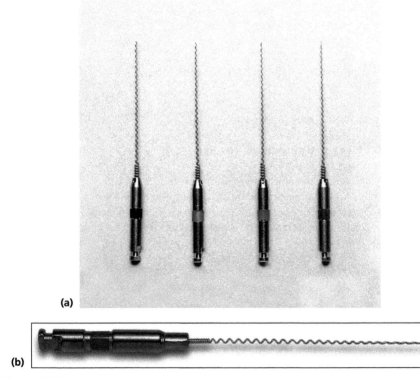

(a)

(b)

Figure 10.8

FIGURE 10.7

Name
Disposable irrigating syringe and disposable needle

Function, features and precaution
- Used with an irrigant to clean and disinfect the canal during endodontic treatment
- A blunt needle with side exiting delivery will reduce the risk of the needle binding within the canal
- Size of syringe and needle vary depending on operator preference
- Needle to be disposed of in the sharps' container and are single use

Varieties
Locking type: assists in prevention of splashing and needle displacement

FIGURE 10.8a, b

Name
Lentulo spiral filler/rotary paste filler

Function and features
- Small flexible instrument used to place materials into the canal
- Fits into the conventional handpiece
- Use with caution as it can be easily broken
- Different sizes available
- Disposed of in the sharps' container and are single use

INSTRUMENTS USED IN
ENDODONTIC TREATMENT

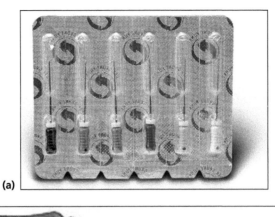

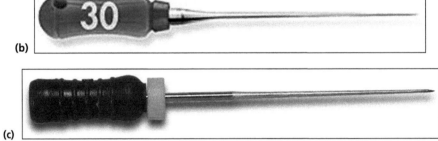

Figure 10.9

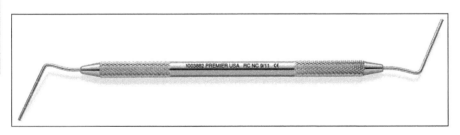

Figure 10.10

FIGURE 10.9a, b

Name
Finger spreader

Function, features and precaution
- Used to condense gutta percha into the canal during obturation
- Finger instrument with a smooth, pointed, tapered working end
- Disposed of in the sharps' container

Varieties
Can be of the hand instrument type (lateral condenser)

False friends
Endodontic K files, Hedström files, barbed broaches

FIGURE 10.10

Name
Endodontic plugger

Function
Working end is flat to facilitate plugging or condensing the gutta percha after the excess has been removed by melting off with a heated instrument

Varieties
- Different sizes of working ends are available
- Available as hand or finger instruments

INSTRUMENTS USED IN
ENDODONTIC TREATMENT

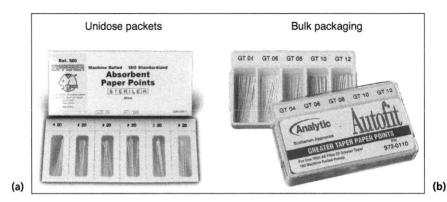

Figure 10.11

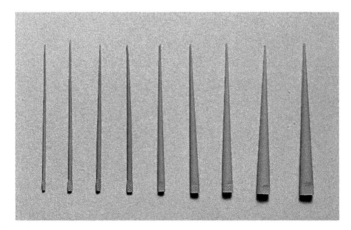

Figure 10.12

ENDODONTIC ACCESSORIES

FIGURE 10.11a, b, c

Name
Absorbent paper points

Functions
- To absorb any moisture in the canal (i.e. blood, pus and saliva)
- To carry medicaments into the canal

Varieties
Can be packaged in unidose (sterile) or bulk packaging (once package is open they are not sterile)

FIGURE 10.12

Name
Gutta percha points

Function and features
- Non-soluble, non-irritant points that are condensed into the pulp chamber during obturation
- Standardised type: follows same ISO classification as endodontic files
- Non-standardised: have a greater taper than the standard ISO type

Varieties
- Can be packaged in single dose or bulk packages
- Different sizes with different tapers available

INSTRUMENTS USED IN
ENDODONTIC TREATMENT

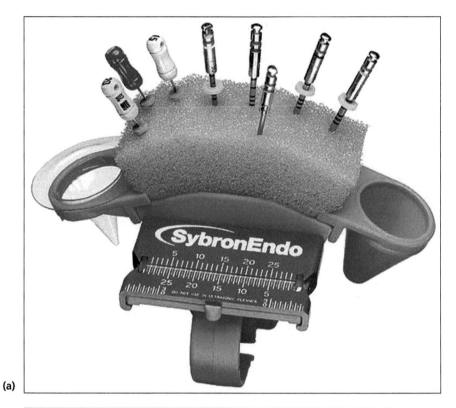

(a)

(b)

Figure 10.13

FIGURES 10.13a, b; 10.14a, b

Name
(Figure 10.13a) Endodontic ring (Figure 10.13b) Endodontic block (Figure 10.14 a, b) Endodontic rulers

Functions
- An endodontic block is a sturdy block used to organise and hold endodontic finger and rotary instruments during procedures; allows easy and accurate measurement of the length of finger instruments (measuring device incorporated)
- Reduces the possibility of percutaneous injuries when handling endodontic finger and rotary instruments
- Special endodontic rulers are available for measuring the length of finger instruments

Varieties
Different varieties available

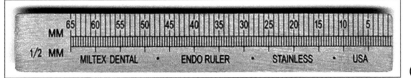

(a)

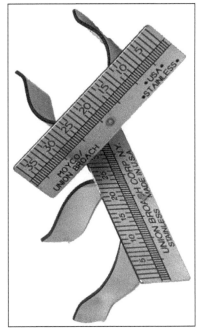

Figure 10.14

(b)

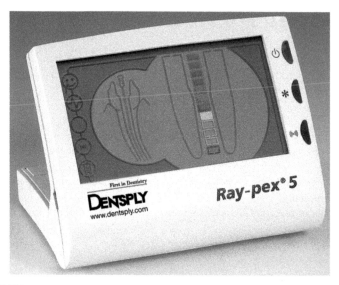

Figure 10.15

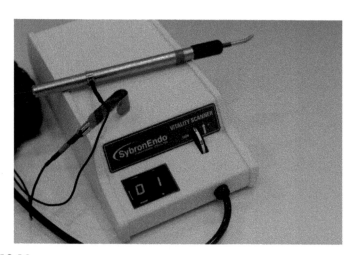

Figure 10.16

FIGURE 10.15

Name
Apex locator

Functions
- An electronic instrument used to determine the distance to the apical foramen
- The screen allows the operator to visualise the file movement during instrumentation

Varieties
- Different manufacturers provide different varieties
- Available with a pulp tester incorporated in the machine

FIGURE 10.16

Name
Electric pulp tester

Function and directions for use
- Used to test the vitality of a tooth using electric stimulus
- Electric stimulus is increased in small increments until the patient can feel the stimulus
- Toothpaste or prophy paste is used to conduct the current from the pulp tester to the tooth

Varieties
- Available with an apex locator incorporated in the machine
- Different manufacturers supply different varieties of pulp testers
- Can use a cold substance to test the vitality of the pulp, i.e. ethyl chloride or Endo Cold Spray

INSTRUMENTS USED IN
ENDODONTIC TREATMENT

Set-ups

The following instruments are common to all the below listed set-ups:
- Mouth mirror and handle (p. 34, 35)
- Sickle/contra-angled probe (p. 36, 37)
- College tweezers (locking type optional) (p. 39, 40)
- High and low volume/disposable saliva ejector suction tips (p. 42, 43)
- Instruments for local anaesthetic set-up (see Section 5, p. 49)
- Instruments for rubber dam set-up (see Section 6, p. 61)
- Sterile cotton pellets (p. 44, 45)
- Air turbine handpiece (p. 70, 71)
- Conventional handpiece (p. 74, 75)
- Various burs (see Section 7, p. 69)
- Radiographs and appropriate film and holders (suitable for use with the rubber dam and clamp in position) (see Section 2, p. 15)

Root canal treatment (first appointment is the same as a pulpectomy): removal of the pulp, cleaning and disinfection of the canal and obturation (may take multiple visits).
- DG16 probe/endodontic probe
- Barbed broaches
- Gates Glidden drills
- Endodontic K files
- Ruler
- Spiral fillers
- Finger spreaders
- Irrigation syringe, needle and irrigation fluid
- Paper points
- Gutta percha and heat source
- Mortonson-Clevedent plugger (p. 96, 97)
- Sealing material and desired filling material (temporary or permanent)

Pulpotomy: removal of the infected or exposed portion of the pulp.
- Calcium hydroxide
- Temporary filling material

Apicectomy: may be needed when root canal treatment has failed. Involves removal of the infected apex and the surrounding infection and replacement with desired filling material.
- Sterile bib and barriers
- Surgical suction tip
- Scalpel handle and disposable scalpel blade (pp. 174 and 175)
- Periosteal elevator, surgical curette
- Spoon excavator (p. 88, 89)
- Straight handpiece and burs (see Section 7, p. 72, 73)
- Ultrasonic unit with appropriate tip (p. 264, 265)
- Irrigation syringe, needle, irrigant (saline) and galley pot
- Desired filling material, mixing slab, messing gun, small pluggers and a burnisher
- Set-up for suturing (see Section 13, p. 169)

INSTRUMENTS USED IN
ENDODONTIC TREATMENT

SECTION 11
ELEVATORS

Elevators are used to loosen and 'elevate' the teeth in their sockets prior to extraction. Care needs to be taken when using elevators to avoid causing trauma to the adjacent teeth.

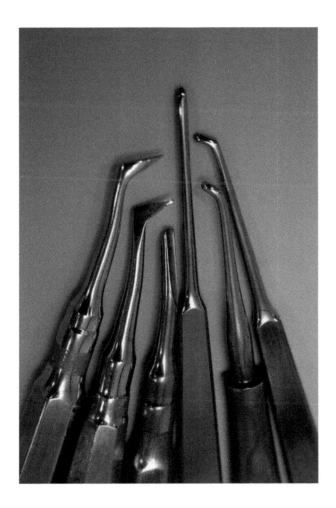

Basic Guide to Dental Instruments, Second Edition. Carmen Scheller-Sheridan.
© 2011 Carmen Scheller-Sheridan. Published 2011 by Blackwell Publishing Ltd.

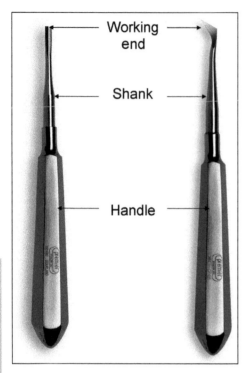

Working end

Shank

Handle

Figure 11.1

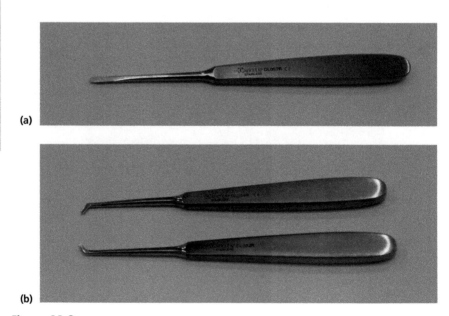

(a)

(b)

Figure 11.2

PARTS OF AN ELEVATOR

FIGURE 11.1

Working end
- The working end is the functional, elevating and retracting end of the elevator
- Single-ended
- The working end is adapted to the function of the instrument

Shank
- The area between the working end and the handle
- The shank may be straight or angled for easy access to some areas in the mouth
- The shank may also have a finger rest to enable the operator to get a better grip and apply more force

Handle
- The part of the instrument that the operator holds
- Designed for stability and leverage
- The handle can be of many different varieties (i.e. serrated, smooth, hollow, solid, octagonal, round, large and small)
- The function dictates the type of handle

TYPES OF ELEVATOR

FIGURE 11.2a, b

Name
(a) Warwick James elevator – straight (b) Warwick James elevators – left and right

Family
Elevators

Function and features
- Used to elevate and loosen the tooth from the periodontal ligament
- Elevation is done to create space and prevent trauma to adjacent teeth and tissues
- Available as left and right elevators, designed to adapt to the mesial and distal aspects of the tooth, respectively.
- Always used as a pair

False friends
Couplands chisel, Mershon band pusher

ELEVATORS

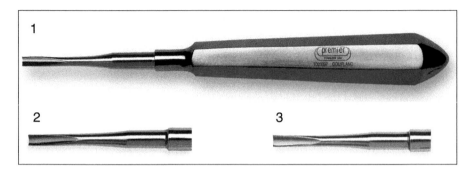

Figure 11.3

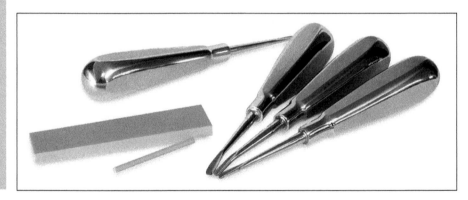

Figure 11.4

FIGURE 11.3

Name
Couplands chisel

Family
Elevators

Function and types
- Used to elevate and loosen the tooth from the periodontal ligament
- Elevation is done to create space and prevent trauma to adjacent teeth and tissues
- Available in sizes 1, 2 and 3 – working end gets larger with increase in size number

False friends
Warwick James straight elevator, Warwick James left and right elevators, Mershon band pusher

FIGURE 11.4

Name
Luxator/Luxating elevator

Family
Elevators

Function and types
- Used to elevate and loosen the tooth from the periodontal ligament
- Elevation is done to create space and prevent trauma to adjacent teeth and tissues

False friends
Warwick James straight elevator, Warwick James left and right elevators, Mershon band pusher

ELEVATORS

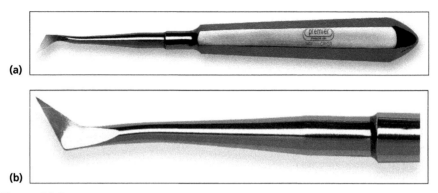

(a)

(b)

Figure 11.5

FIGURE 11.5a, b

Name

Cryers elevators – left and right (Enlarged working end Figure 11.4b)

Family

Elevators

Functions

- Used to remove interseptal bone
- Used to loosen root tips

Set-up

- Elevators are always used in conjunction with other dental instruments
- Please see set-ups in Sections 12 and 13 (p. 155, 169)

ELEVATORS

SECTION 12
EXTRACTION FORCEPS

Extraction forceps are used along with elevators to extract teeth. Each extraction forcep is designed for a particular area of the mouth. The beaks are designed to fit around the cervical portion of the tooth. Pointed beaks are designed to grip the furcation area.

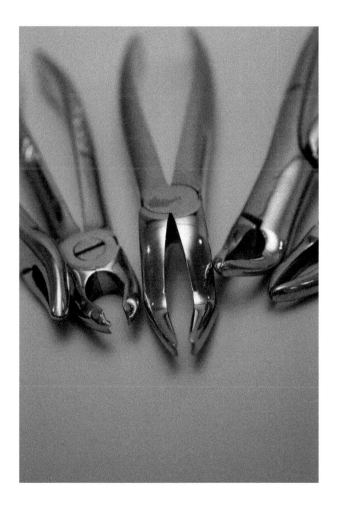

Basic Guide to Dental Instruments, Second Edition. Carmen Scheller-Sheridan.
© 2011 Carmen Scheller-Sheridan. Published 2011 by Blackwell Publishing Ltd.

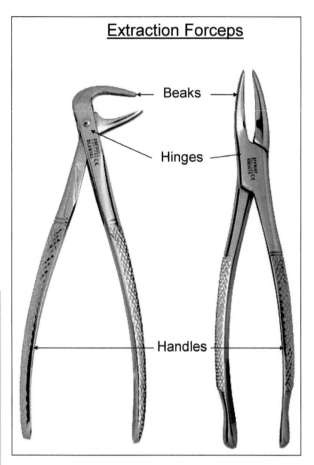

Extraction Forceps

Beaks

Hinges

Handles

Figure 12.1

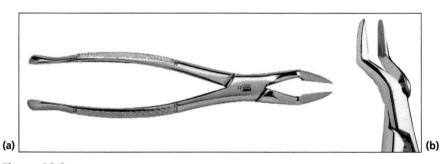

(a)

(b)

Figure 12.2

PARTS OF EXTRACTION FORCEPS

FIGURE 12.1

Beak
- The beaks of extraction forceps are designed to fit around the curve of the tooth's crown
- Universal forceps have a beak that can be used in any quadrant of the mouth
- Forceps designed for multi-rooted teeth have beaks with a point that is adapted to grip the tooth furcation
- Forceps designed for single-rooted teeth usually have smooth beaks

Hinge
- Extraction forceps have hinges (can be screw or pin type) allowing the beak and handle to be opened and grasped
- Care must be taken with hinges to prevent damage during sterilisation (see manufacturer's instructions for appropriate care)

Handle
- A serrated handle allows the operator to have a better grip
- A palm grasp is used with the handle of extraction forceps
- A curve on the end of the handle may be present for the little finger, to provide more stability and leverage
- Handles of maxillary forceps are often curved upwards, with the beak in line with the handle
- Mandibular forceps tend to have a straight handle with the beak at a 90° angle to the handle

TYPES OF EXTRACTION FORCEPS

FIGURE 12.2a, b

Name
Bayonet extraction forceps

Family
Extraction forceps

Function
Elongated beak is designed for extraction of maxillary third molars and roots

EXTRACTION FORCEPS

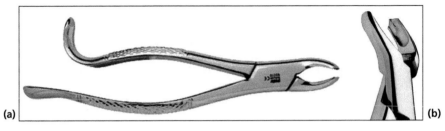

Figure 12.3

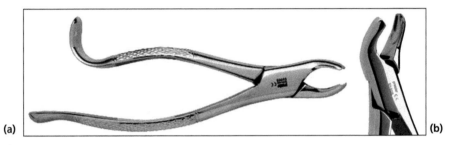

Figure 12.4

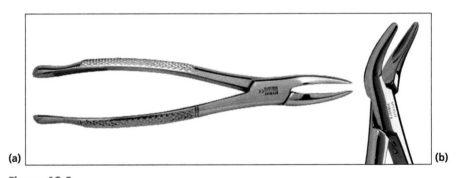

Figure 12.5

FIGURE 12.3a, b

Name
Maxillary right permanent molar extraction forceps

Family
Extraction forceps

Function
Used for extraction of maxillary right permanent molar teeth

Identifying features
To determine whether left or right forceps:
- Hold forceps in hand loosely (beak facing patient)
- The point of the beak should grip the furcation on the buccal side ('beak to cheek')

False friend
Maxillary left permanent molar extraction forceps

FIGURE 12.4a, b

Name
Maxillary left permanent molar extraction forceps

Family
Extraction forceps

Function
Used for extraction of maxillary left permanent molar teeth

Identifying features
To determine whether left or right forceps:
- Hold forceps in hand loosely (beak facing patient)
- The point of the beak should grip the furcation on the buccal side ('beak to cheek')

False friend
Maxillary right permanent molar extraction forceps

FIGURE 12.5a, b

Name
Maxillary root extraction forceps

Family
Extraction forceps

Function
The extended beak is designed for extraction of maxillary roots

EXTRACTION FORCEPS

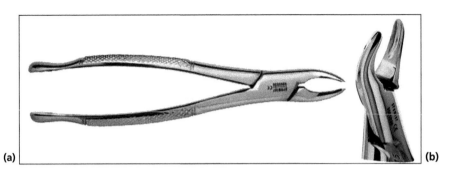

Figure 12.6

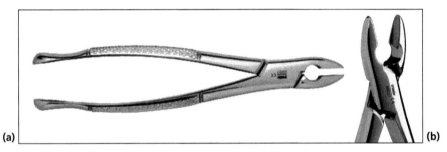

Figure 12.7

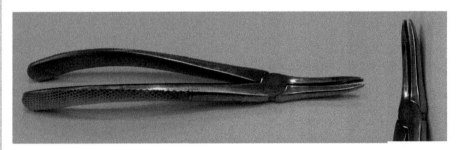

Figure 12.8

EXTRACTION FORCEPS

FIGURE 12.6a, b

Name
Maxillary premolar extraction forceps

Family
Extraction forceps

Function
Used for extraction of maxillary permanent canines, premolars and anterior deciduous teeth

False friend
Maxillary permanent straight extraction forceps

FIGURE 12.7a, b

Name
Maxillary straight extraction forceps/maxillary permanent incisor extraction forceps. Also called: maxillary permanent anterior extraction forceps

Family
Extraction forceps

Function
Used for extraction of maxillary anterior permanent teeth. Smaller version available for extraction of maxillary deciduous canines

FIGURE 12.8

Name
Greyhound extraction forceps. Also called: maxillary root extraction forceps

Family
Extraction forceps

Function
Used for extraction of maxillary roots

EXTRACTION FORCEPS

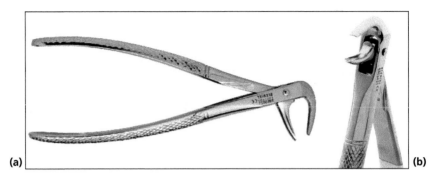

(a)   (b)

Figure 12.9

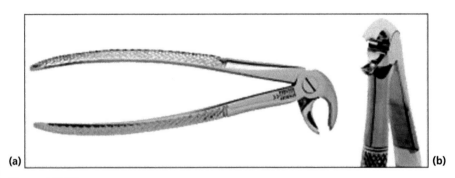

(a)   (b)

Figure 12.10

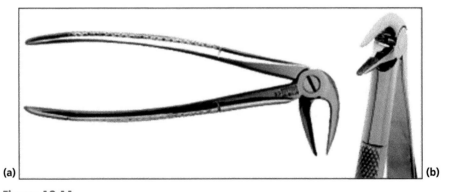

(a)   (b)

Figure 12.11

FIGURE 12.9a, b

Name
Mandibular permanent premolar extraction forceps

Family
Extraction forceps

Function
- Used for extraction of mandibular permanent anterior and premolar teeth
- Can be used on mandibular right or left side

False friends
Mandibular root forceps

FIGURE 12.10a, b

Name
Mandibular permanent molar extraction forceps

Family
Extraction forceps

Function and feature
- Used for extraction of mandibular permanent teeth
- Point of the beak fits in the furcation of the molars
- Can be used on mandibular right or left side

False friend
Mandibular deciduous molar extraction forceps

FIGURE 12.11a, b

Name
Mandibular root extraction forceps

Family
Extraction forceps

Function
- Used for extraction of permanent mandibular roots
- Can be used on mandibular right or left side

EXTRACTION FORCEPS

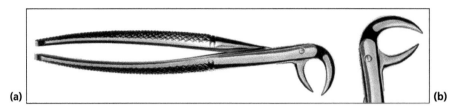

(a)   (b)

Figure 12.12

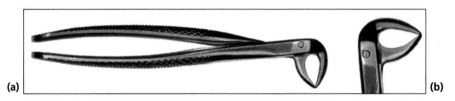

(a)   (b)

Figure 12.13

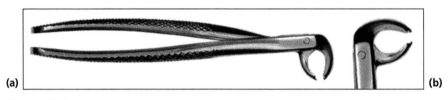

(a)   (b)

Figure 12.14

EXTRACTION FORCEPS

FIGURE 12.12a, b

Name
Cowhorn extraction forceps

Family
Extraction forceps

Function and features
- Used for extraction of mandibular permanent molars
- Point of the beak is designed to grip the furcation of the molars
- Can be used on the mandibular right or left side

FIGURE 12.13a, b

Name
Mandibular deciduous anterior extraction forceps

Family
Extraction forceps

Functions
- Used for extraction of mandibular deciduous anterior teeth
- Can be used on mandibular right or left side

FIGURE 12.14a, b

Name
Mandibular deciduous posterior extraction forceps

Family
Extraction forceps

Functions
- Used for extraction of deciduous mandibular posterior teeth

EXTRACTION FORCEPS

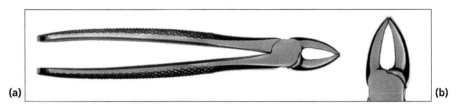

(a)   (b)

Figure 12.15

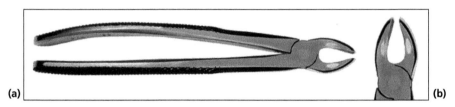

(a)   (b)

Figure 12.16

EXTRACTION FORCEPS

FIGURE 12.15a, b

Name
Maxillary deciduous molar extraction forceps

Family
Extraction forceps

Functions
- Used for extraction of deciduous maxillary molar teeth
- Can be used on maxillary right or left side

FIGURE 12.16a, b

Name
Mandibular deciduous molar extraction forceps

Family
Extraction forceps

Functions
- Used for extraction of deciduous mandibular molar teeth
- Can be used to extract small permanent third molars
- Can be used on mandibular right or left side

EXTRACTION FORCEPS

Set-ups

The following instruments are common to all the below listed set-ups:
- Mouth mirror and handle (p. 34, 35)
- Sickle/contra-angled probe (p. 36, 37)
- College tweezers (p. 39, 40)
- Instruments for local anaesthetic set-up (see Section 5, p. 49)

Routine extractions
- High and low volume/disposable saliva ejector suction tips (p. 42, 43)
- Periosteal elevator (p. 174, 175)
- Couplands chisel (p. 150, 151)
- Operator's choice of forceps and elevators

Surgical extractions
- Sterile bib and barriers
- Surgical suction (p. 180, 181)
- McKesson mouth prop (p. 170, 171)
- Scalpel handle and disposable scalpel blade (pp. 174 and 175)
- Periosteal elevator (p. 174, 175)
- Bowdler Henry rake, Kilner or Austin retractor (p. 172, 173)
- Irrigation syringe, disposable needle and irrigant (p. 136, 137)
- Galley pot (p. 188, 189)
- Straight handpiece (p. 72, 73)
- Various burs (see Section 7, p. 69)
- Couplands chisel (p. 150, 151)
- Warwick James left and right elevators (p. 148, 149)
- Warwick James straight elevator (p. 148, 149)
- Surgical curette (p. 176, 177)
- Bone file (p. 180, 181)
- Operator's choice of extraction forceps
- Suturing set-up (see Section 13, p. 169)
- Sterile gauze, bib and barriers
- Post-operative instruction sheet

SECTION 13
SURGICAL INSTRUMENTS

Many procedures may involve an invasive surgical approach, requiring special dental instruments. Due to the specialised nature of this area, some of these instruments may not be used in the general dental surgery, and some of these procedures may be carried out in conjunction with various sedation techniques. It is important that during these procedures the dental team tries to maintain the most sterile field possible.

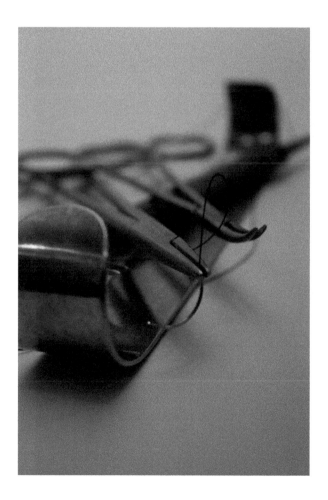

Basic Guide to Dental Instruments, Second Edition. Carmen Scheller-Sheridan.
© 2011 Carmen Scheller-Sheridan. Published 2011 by Blackwell Publishing Ltd.

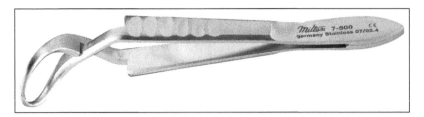

Figure 13.1

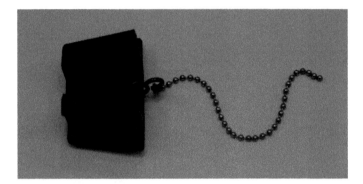

Figure 13.2

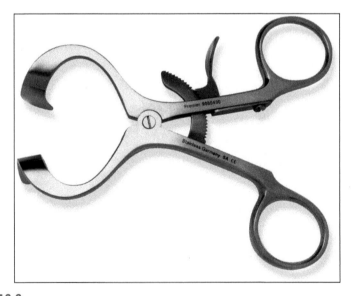

Figure 13.3

GENERAL SURGICAL INSTRUMENTS

FIGURE 13.1

Name
Towel clip

Function
Used to secure bibs and towels in place

Varieties
Various sizes and shapes available

FIGURE 13.2

Name
McKesson mouth prop

Function and feature
• Used to prop open mouth
• Attached to a parachute chain for retrieval in case of displacement (made of rubber to protect teeth)

Varieties
• Various colours and shapes available
• Available in small, medium and large sizes, or sizes 1, 2 and 3

FIGURE 13.3

Name
Mouth spreader/gag

Functions
• Used to prop open mouth
• A locking mechanism on handle props open the mouth
• Can be used during sedation procedures

Varieties
Various sizes and shapes available

SURGICAL INSTRUMENTS

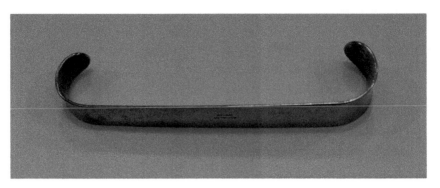

Figure 13.4

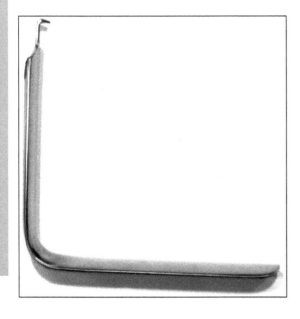

Figure 13.5

FIGURE 13.4

Name
Kilner cheek retractor

Functions
- Retraction of cheek
- Aids in visibility
- Protection of tissues

FIGURE 13.5

Name
Austin retractor

Functions
- Aids in visibility
- Protection of tissues
- Retraction of cheek and tongue

FIGURE 13.6

Name
Bowdler Henry rake retractor

Functions
- Retraction of periodontal flap during surgical procedures
- Aids in visibility
- Protection of tissues

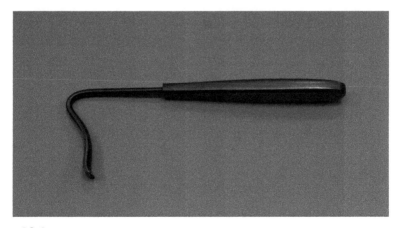

Figure 13.6

SURGICAL INSTRUMENTS

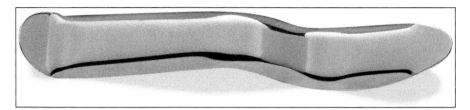

Figure 13.7

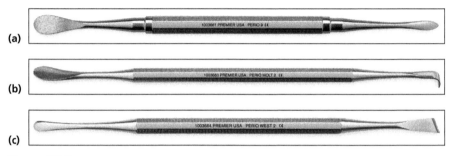

(a)

(b)

(c)

Figure 13.8

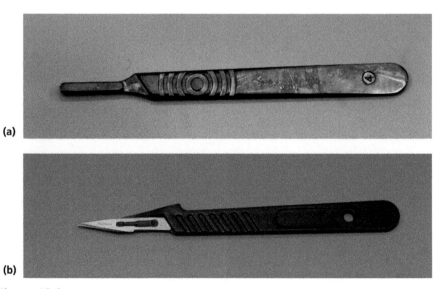

(a)

(b)

Figure 13.9

FIGURE 13.7

Name
Minnesota retractor

Functions
- Aids in visibility
- Protection of tissues
- Retraction of the cheek and tongue

Varieties
Different varieties of retractors available

FIGURE 13.8a, b, c

Name
Howarths periosteal elevator

Family
Elevators

Functions and features
- Retraction
- To separate the tissue from the bone
- One working end is a pointed tip and the other is rounded with sharp edges

Varieties
Different lengths and shapes of working ends available

False friend
Bone file

FIGURE 13.9a, b

Name
(a) Stainless steel scalpel handle (b) Disposable scalpel handle and scalpel blade

Functions and features
- Scalpel handle holds disposable scalpel blade securely
- Surgical blade used to make incisions intra-orally
- Stainless steel scalpel handle – autoclavable

Varieties
- Can have a plastic scalpel handle – disposable
- Various sizes and shapes of scalpel blades available

SURGICAL INSTRUMENTS

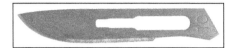

Figure 13.10

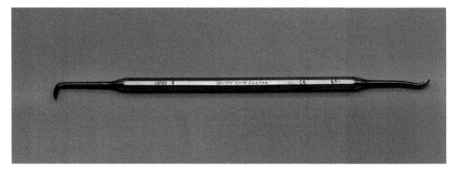

Figure 13.11

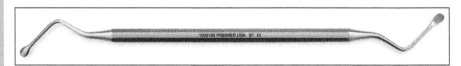

Figure 13.12

FIGURE 13.10

Name
Disposable scalpel blade

Function and features
- Scalpel blades are used to make incisions
- Made of surgical carbon steel
- Different shapes for different procedures (e.g. 11 blade and 15 blade)
- Single use
- Disposed of in the sharps' container
- Supplied in a sterile package

Varieties
Available in different shapes, sizes and lengths depending on procedure

FIGURE 13.11

Name
Mitchells trimmer

Functions
- To aid in raising the mucoperiosteal flap for access
- To aid in removing pathology

False friend
Wards carver

FIGURE 13.12

Name
Spoon curette/surgical curette

Function
Used in the socket of an extracted tooth to remove debris and infectious material

Variations
Shank can be straight, curved or shaped like a spoon, with different sizes of working ends

False friend
Spoon excavator

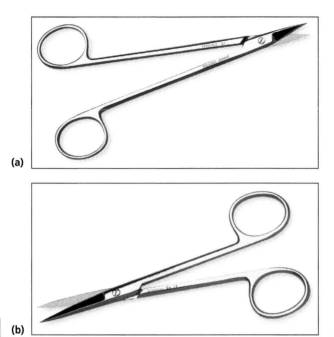

(a)

(b)

Figure 13.13

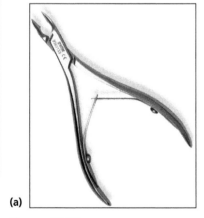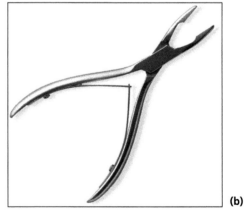

(a)   (b)

Figure 13.14

FIGURE 13.13a, b

Name
(a) Curved surgical scissors (b) Straight surgical scissors

Function
Sharp pointed scissors are used for cutting soft tissues in surgical procedures

Variations
- Different lengths and sizes available
- Working ends can be curved or straight

False friends
Suture scissors, blunt scissors

FIGURE 13.14a, b

Name
(a) Bone rongeurs (b) Bone nibblers

Function and features
- Used to trim sharp edges of bone remaining after extractions
- Usually used during multiple extractions
- Have a spring mechanism between the handles
- Have a sharpened working end
- Can be end-cutting or side-cutting
- Can be used in any quadrant in the mouth

False friend
Extraction forceps

SURGICAL INSTRUMENTS

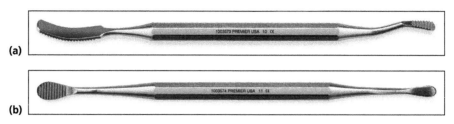

(a)

(b)

Figure 13.15

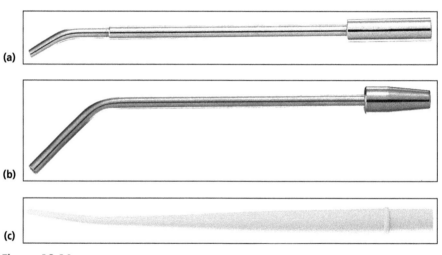

(a)

(b)

(c)

Figure 13.16

FIGURE 13.15a, b

Name
Bone file

Function and direction for use
- Used to remove and smooth sharp pieces of alveolar bone remaining after extraction
- Used with a push–pull action

False friend
Periosteal elevator

FIGURE 13.16a, b, c

Name
(a, b) Metal autoclavable surgical suction tips (c) Plastic disposable surgical suction tip

Function
For suction in surgical procedures

Varieties
- Different sizes and shapes available
- Can be made of metal, plastic or sterile disposable plastic

SURGICAL INSTRUMENTS

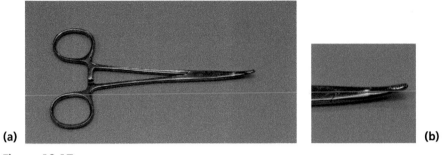

(a)   (b)

Figure 13.17

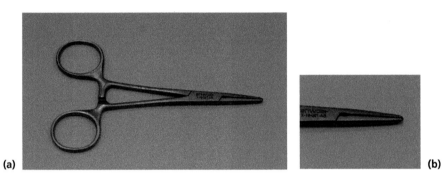

(a)   (b)

Figure 13.18

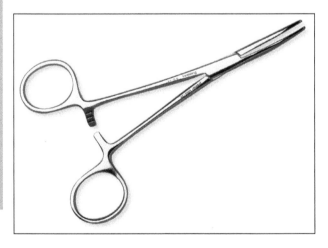

Figure 13.19

FIGURES 13.17a, b; 13.18a, b; 13.19

Name
(Figure 13.17a, b) Mosquito artery forceps – straight (Figure 13.18a, b) Mosquito artery forceps – curved (Figure 13.19) Haemostat

Functions and features
- Used for grasping objects and holding them securely
- Can be used to apply pressure to a severed artery
- Handle has a locking mechanism

Varieties
- Many different sizes available
- Working end angle can vary

False friends
Beebee crown scissors, needle holders

FIGURE 13.20a, b

Name
(a) Mayo needle holder (b) Castroviejo needle holder

Function and feature
- Used along with tissue dissecting forceps during suturing
- Locking mechanism on the handle holds suture securely while suturing
- Scissor-like surgical instrument with serrated edges for better grip

Varieties
Many different shapes and sizes available

False friends
Mosquito artery forceps, suture scissors, surgical scissors, haemostats

SURGICAL INSTRUMENTS

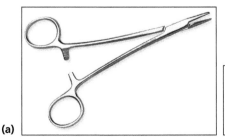

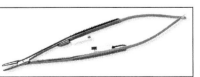

(a)   (b)

Figure 13.20

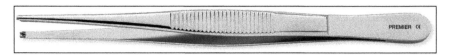

Figure 13.21

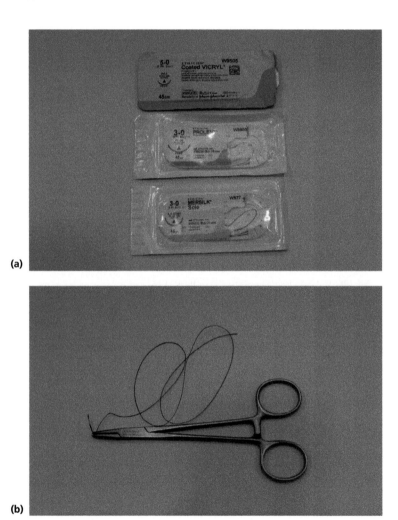

(a)

(b)

Figure 13.22

FIGURE 13.21

Name
Toothed dissecting forceps/tissue dissecting forceps

Functions and feature
- Used to retract tissues, 'teeth' on working end aid in grasping tissue
- Facilitate suturing

False friend
College tweezers

FIGURE 13.22a, b

Name
Various sutures

Function and features
- Aid in healing by closing tissue after surgery
- Pre-threaded disposable suture needles
- Supplied sterile in a package
- Suture needles are curved with a sharp edge

Varieties
- Many different sizes available
- Can be made of different materials (e.g. silk and absorbable materials)

SURGICAL INSTRUMENTS

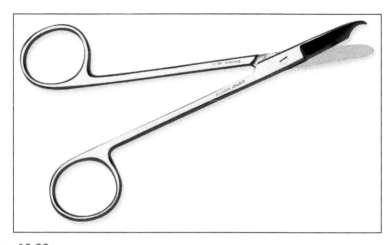

Figure 13.23

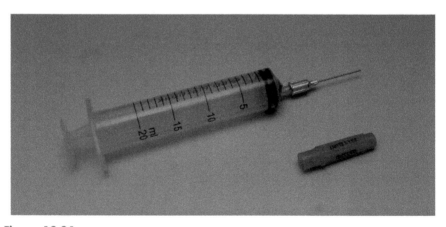

Figure 13.24

FIGURE 13.23

Name
Suture scissors

Function and features
- Scissors designed for suture removal
- Blades – one has a curved edge and one has a notched edge
- During suture removal, suture is scooped up by blade with the notched end before cutting to prevent tissue trauma

False friends
Surgical scissors, needle holders

FIGURE 13.24

Name
(a) Disposable irrigating syringe and disposable needle (b) Assembled disposable irrigation syringe and disposable needle

Function and precaution
- Used in conjunction with saline solution to provide water spray when using handpiece during a surgical procedure
- Used to irrigate and rinse treatment area
- Should be used with a blunt needle to prevent injury

Varieties
- Locking type – prevents splashing and needle displacement
- Size of syringe and needle vary depending on operator preference

SURGICAL INSTRUMENTS

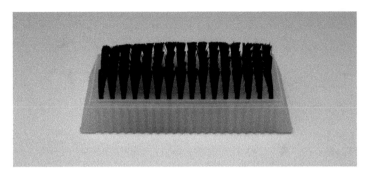

Figure 13.25

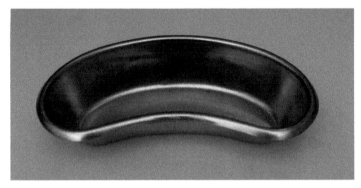

Figure 13.26

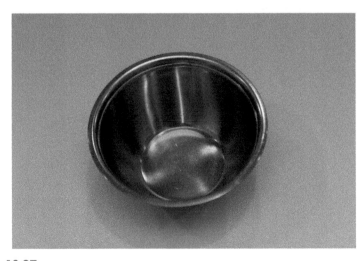

Figure 13.27

FIGURE 13.25

Name
Nail brush

Function and precaution
- Used to clean under fingernails during a surgical scrub
- Surgical scrub technique should be followed according to the local infection control policy

Varieties
Different sizes and shapes available

FIGURE 13.26

Name
Kidney dish

Functions
- Used to hold instruments when preparing for a surgical procedure
- Used to hold liquids or materials
- Used if patient gets ill

Varieties
- Many different sizes and shapes
- Available in disposable or metal types

FIGURE 13.27

Name
Galley pot

Function
Used to hold saline for irrigation

Varieties
Various sizes available

SURGICAL INSTRUMENTS

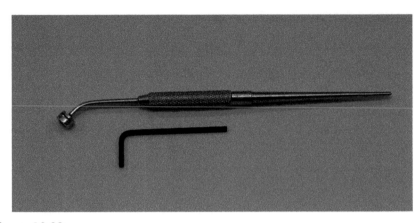

Figure 13.28

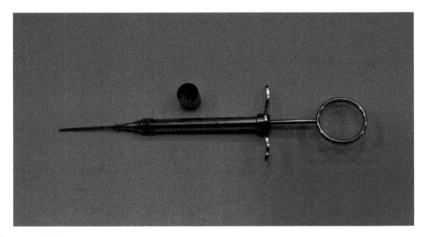

Figure 13.29

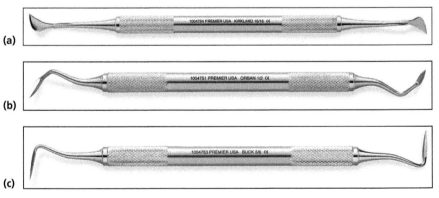

(a)

(b)

(c)

Figure 13.30

INSTRUMENTS FOR PERIODONTAL SURGERY

FIGURE 13.28

Name
Blake's gingivectomy knife handle

Function and features
- A handle designed specifically to grasp a disposable scalpel blade for cutting gingival tissue
- Allen key provided to secure blade to handle

Varieties
Can be used with different sizes and shapes of blades

FIGURE 13.29

Name
Messing gun

Function and description
- Modified and specialised amalgam carrier
- Used in retrograde filling procedure (of a root apex)
- Used during apiceoctomy

False friend
Amalgam carrier

FIGURE 13.30a, b, c

Name
(a) Gingivectomy knives (b) Kirkland (c) Orban Goldman-Fox Buck

Function
Used to contour and incise gingival tissue during periodontal surgery

Varieties
Various sizes available

SURGICAL INSTRUMENTS

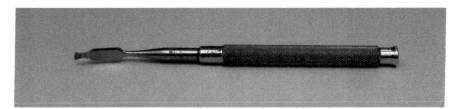

Figure 13.31

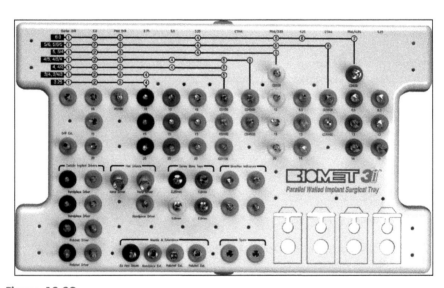

Figure 13.32

SURGICAL INSTRUMENTS

FIGURE 13.31

Name
Ochsenbein chisel

Function, features and direction for use
• Used to remove and smooth areas of the bone during surgical procedures
• Working end is a flat bevelled cutting blade
• Used with a small broad push stroke

Varieties
Various sizes available

IMPLANTS

A dental implant is a surgically placed device which is placed in the maxilla or mandible, which in conjunction with a prosthesis replaces a missing tooth or teeth. The implant replaces the root of the tooth and supports a crown, bridge or denture with the purpose of replacing the missing tooth/teeth.

FIGURE 13.32

Name
Implant kit

Function and features
• Used in conjunction with the placement of dental implants
• Specialised drills used in conjunction with implant procedures
• Drills may be colour coded for easy identification
• Requires a special conventional handpiece
• Sterile technique must be practiced during dental implant placements
• Implant systems vary between dental suppliers

Varieties
Many different types of drills and kits available

SURGICAL INSTRUMENTS

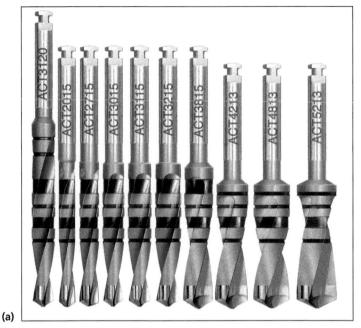
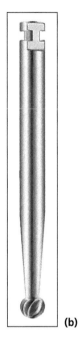

(a)   (b)

Figure 13.33

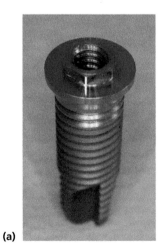
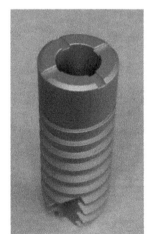

(a)   (b)

Figure 13.34

FIGURE 13.33a, b

Name
Implant drills

Function and features
- Various drills are used for preparation of the implant placement site
- Small round drill increasing in size and moving to twist drills
- Prepared implant placement site is slightly smaller than the size of the dental implant to be placed
- Use of burs and drills during dental implant placement is done using copious amounts of water

Varieties
Many different types of drills available

FIGURE 13.34 (a) External connection – Biomet 3i and (b) Internal connection – Ankylos

Name
Implant/screw/fixture/post

Function and features
- A 'screw' which is surgically inserted into the maxillary or mandibular arch which acts as a replacement for the natural root of a tooth or teeth
- Surfaces are designed for osseointegration
- Available in various diameters and lengths which correspond to the size and length of the tooth to be replaced
- The 'top' or cervical portion of the dental implant is referred to the platform, where the cover screw, healing abutment and final abutment seat
- The platform of the implant is available as an external (protruding) connection or an internal (screw access hole) connection which may be shaped in hexagonal, triangle or tapered cone shapes
- Each implant has a screw access hole that is accessed from the platform and receives the cover screw, healing abutment and final abutment

Varieties
Vary depending on operator preference, use and manufacturer

SURGICAL INSTRUMENTS

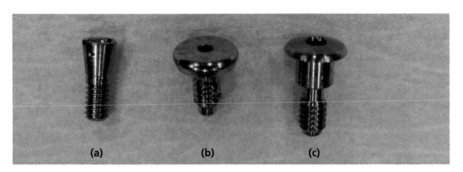

Figure 13.35

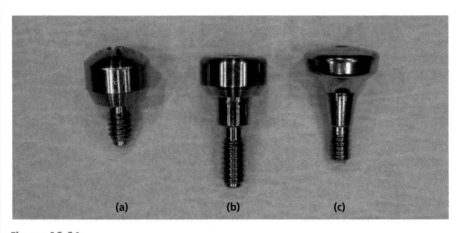

Figure 13.36

FIGURE 13.35 (a) Ankylos, (b) Biomet 3i and (c) Nobel Biocare

Name
Cover screw

Function and features
- A screw which threads into the screw access hole, covering the platform and connection (screwed into the screw access hole) of the dental implant immediately after placement
- Its function is to protect the dental implant and sealing it from debris, bone and gingiva during the healing and integration period
- The cover screw projects approximately 1 mm above the platform of implant, and during the integration period is covered by the soft tissues
- The cover screw is normally in place for approximately 3–4 months
- The cover screw is surgically removed during the next stage of implant placement and replaced with a healing abutment

Varieties
Vary depending on manufacturer

FIGURE 13.36 (a) Biomet 3i, (b) Nobel Biocare and (c) Ankylos

Name
Healing abutment/healing cap/sulcus former

Function and features
- Its function is to protect the dental implant, sealing it from debris, bone and gingiva during the healing process
- The healing abutment screws into the screw access hole and fits the platform of the implant
- It projects above the gingiva, leaving it exposed in the mouth
- Available in different heights

Varieties
Vary depending on manufacturer

SURGICAL INSTRUMENTS

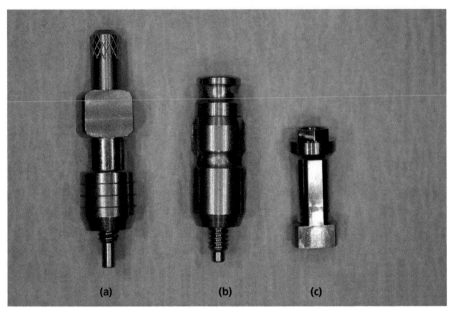

Figure 13.37

FIGURE 13.37a

Name
Pick up (impression) coping

Function and features
- Used with the open tray technique for impression
- Once impression material sets, the retaining screw is loosened allowing the coping to be removed with the impression
- An analogue is fitted to the coping prior to the cast being poured
- Most commonly used

FIGURE 13.37b

Name
Transfer (impression) coping

Function and features
- Used with a closed impression tray
- The impression is removed from the mouth and the coping remains screwed to the implant
- After removal of the impression the coping is removed and placed into the impression
- An analogue is fitted to the coping prior to the cast being poured
- Used in circumstances where patients have limited opening

FIGURE 13.37c Nobel Biocare

Name
Implant analogue

Function and features
- A copy or replica of the dental implant
- Used when the impression of the dental implant is being 'poured up' to replicate the position of the implant in the oral cavity to allow the laboratory technician to construct the prosthesis to fit the implant

Varieties
Vary depending on manufacturer

SURGICAL INSTRUMENTS

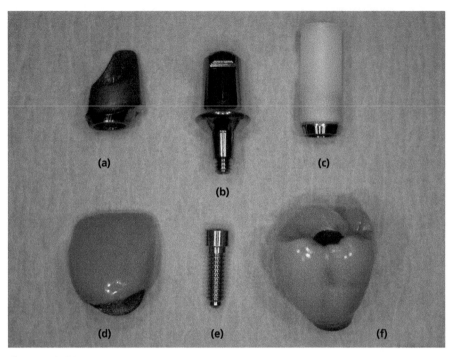

Figure 13.38

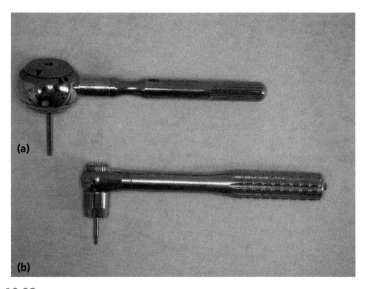

Figure 13.39

FIGURE 13.38 (a) custom abutment – Biomet 3i, (b) stock abutment – Ankylos and (c) UCLA abutment

Name
Abutment

Function and features
- Is used to connect the implant to the prosthetic component
- Prosthetic components may be attached to the abutment either by screw or cementation
- May be temporary, custom made or pre-fabricated
- Abutment type is dependent on the implant chosen

Varieties
Vary depending on manufacturer

FIGURE 13.38 (d) cement retained crown, (e) retaining screw and (f) screw retained crown

Name
Crown

Function and features
- The crown is the portion which is visible in the patient's mouth which resembles a natural tooth

FIGURE 13.39 (a) Biomet 3i and (b) Anklylos

Name
Torque wrench

Function and features
- Used to tighten the retaining screw

SURGICAL INSTRUMENTS

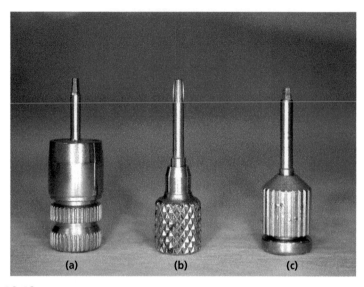

Figure 13.40

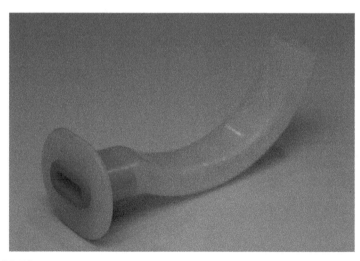

Figure 13.41

FIGURE 13.40 (a) Ankylos, (b) Nobel Biocare and (c) Biomet 3i

Name
Implant driver

Function and features
• Resembles a small screw driver
• Used to fasten and remove cover screws, healing abutment and final abutments retaining screw

EMERGENCY EQUIPMENT

> **!** **This is not meant to be an exhaustive list of emergency equipment that may be needed. These are included in this section due to the nature of surgical procedures.**

FIGURE 13.41

Name
Oro-pharyngeal airway/guedel airway

Function and precautions
• Used in an emergency situation to maintain the patient's airway
• Should be kept in emergency kit
• Must be on premises when conscious sedation is being performed

Varieties
Various sizes available

SURGICAL INSTRUMENTS

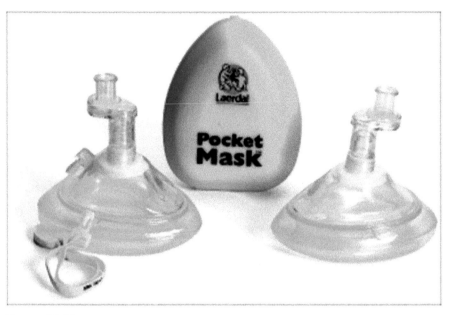

Figure 13.42

FIGURE 13.42

Name

Pocket mask

Function and features

- Used in an emergency situation to provide artificial respiration
- Is fitted with a one-way valve that does not allow fluids to flow between the rescuer and the victim
- Can be used with an oxygen source

Set-ups

The following instruments are common to all the below listed set-ups:
- Mouth mirror and handle (p. 34, 35)
- Sickle/contra-angled probe (p. 36, 37)
- Sterile surgical suction (p. 180, 181)
- Instruments for local anaesthetic set-up (see Section 5, p. 49)

Surgical procedure set-up
- Towel clips
- McKesson mouth props (small, medium or large)
- Sterile gauze, barrier and wrapping
- Sterile surgical gloves
- Kilner cheek retractor, Bowdler Henry rake retractor and Austin retractor
- Scalpel handle and disposable scalpel blade
- Periosteal elevator
- Couplands chisel (standard size 3)
- Warwick James elevators: left, right and straight
- Mitchell trimmer and spoon curette
- Mosquito artery forceps: straight and curved
- Surgical scissors
- Galley pot and kidney dish
- Disposable irrigation syringe and disposable needle
- Straight handpiece and surgical burs
- Bone rongeurs, cutters and nibblers
- Bone file
- Selected sterile sutures
- Toothed dissecting forceps/tissue dissecting forceps
- Mayo needle holder
- Suture scissors
- Post-operative instructions' sheet

Separates
- Extraction forceps (see Section 12, p. 155)

Set-up for suturing
- Pre-threaded sterile suture pack (size and type indicated by operator and procedure)
- Choice of needle holder
- Suture scissors
- Sterile gauze squares
- Toothed dissecting forceps/tissue dissecting forceps

SECTION 14
MEASURING DEVICES

There are many times when instruments are needed for measurement. Some examples of what we may need to measure are: length of root canals, width of lesions and the thickness of crowns.

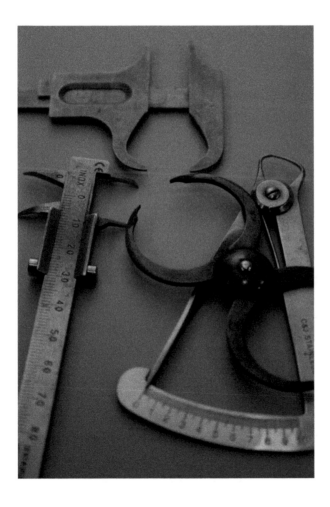

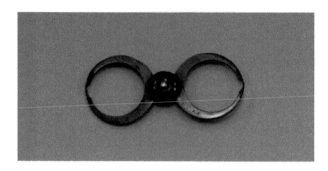

Figure 14.1

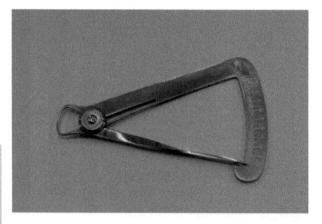

Figure 14.2

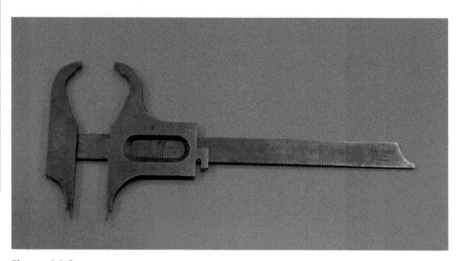

Figure 14.3

FIGURE 14.1

Name
Figure-of-eight calipers

Function and features
- Used for measuring thickness of porcelain and metal
- Calibrated in millimetres and 1/10 millimetre

FIGURE 14.2

Name
Iwanson gauge

Function and features
- Used for measuring thickness of porcelain and metal
- Calibrated in millimetres and 1/10 millimetre

FIGURE 14.3

Name
Boley gauge

Function and features
- Used in the clinic and in the laboratory
- Calibrated in millimetres and 1/10 millimetre

MEASURING DEVICES

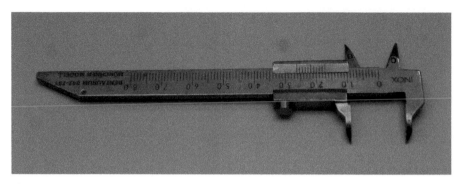

Figure 14.4

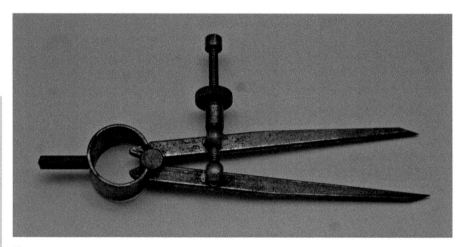

Figure 14.5

MEASURING DEVICES

FIGURE 14.4

Name
Vernier gauge

Function
Used for measuring in many disciplines of dentistry

FIGURE 14.5

Name
Dividers

Function
Used for measuring in many disciplines of dentistry

MEASURING DEVICES

SECTION 15
IMPRESSION TRAYS

Impression trays are used in conjunction with various types of materials to take imprints of the patient's dentition. The type of tray chosen depends on the type of impression needed and the procedure that is indicated.

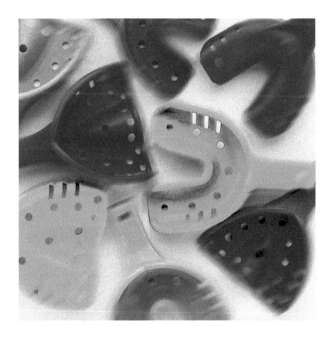

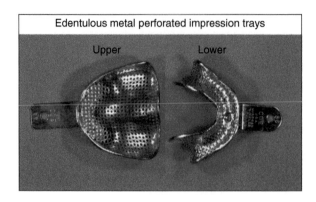

Edentulous metal perforated impression trays

Upper   Lower

Figure 15.1

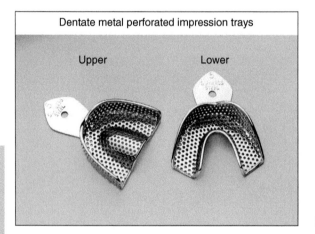

Dentate metal perforated impression trays

Upper   Lower

Figure 15.2

IMPRESSION TRAYS

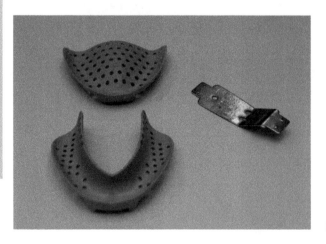

Figure 15.3

FUNCTIONS AND FEATURES OF IMPRESSION TRAYS

- Used to hold impression material
- Can be perforated for better retention
- Have a handle for better grasp during placement and removal
- Dentate impression trays – for patients with teeth
- Edentulous impression trays – for patients with no teeth

TYPES OF IMPRESSION TRAYS

FIGURES 15.1; 15.2

Name
Metal perforated type trays

Features
- Autoclavable
- Available in different sizes (denoted by numbers)
- Not easily adapted
- Available as solid metal trays

FIGURES 15.3; 15.4

Name
Plastic type/stock tray

Features
- Disposable, single use
- A tray adhesive may be used for added retention of impression material
- Available in different sizes (denoted by colours)
- Can be adapted using a heat source

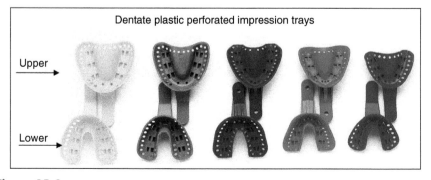

Dentate plastic perforated impression trays

Upper

Lower

Figure 15.4

IMPRESSION TRAYS

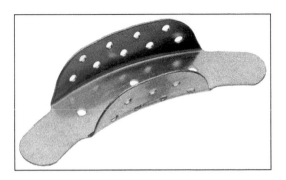

Figure 15.5

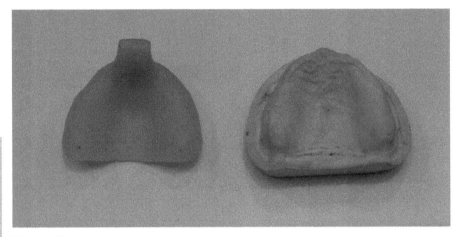

Figure 15.6

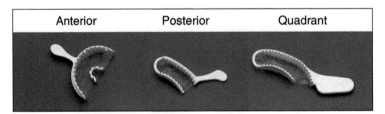

Figure 15.7

IMPRESSION TRAYS

FIGURE 15.5

Name

Universal sectional impression tray

Function and features

- Modified tray used to take an impression of a specific area of the mouth
- May be perforated for retention
- Fabricated from flexible metal – adaptable
- Only suitable for dentate patients
- Autoclavable

FIGURE 15.6

Name

Custom tray/special tray

Features

- Fabricated from a plaster model of the patient's dentate or edentulous arches
- Fabricated from an acrylic material
- Disposable, single use
- Must be 'painted' with tray adhesive for retention of impression material

FIGURE 15.7

Name

Triple tray^{TM}

Function and features

- Used to take an impression of both arches simultaneously
- Fabricated from a combination of plastic and flexible webbing material
- Many different sizes available (anterior, posterior, quadrant)
- Disposable, single use
- Must be painted with tray adhesive for retention of impression material

IMPRESSION TRAYS

Set-up

Set-up for taking an impression. Set-up will vary depending on the type of impression being taken
- Desired impression material
- Desired type of impression tray, tray adhesive and applicator brush
- If required, mixing spatula, mixing bowl and water measure
- Kidney dish – in case of gag reflex when taking impressions (p. 188, 189)
- Tissues and rinse cup for patients
- Wax may be required if the tray needs to be extended
- Laboratory prescription form and laboratory bag
- Red ribbon wax (p. 274, 275)
- Equipment/materials for disinfection of impression prior to sending to the laboratory

IMPRESSION TRAYS

SECTION 16

ORTHODONTIC INSTRUMENTS

Orthodontics is the study of the diagnosis, prevention and treatment of irregularities of the teeth and jaws. Orthodontic instruments are used in conjunction with fixed and removable appliances.

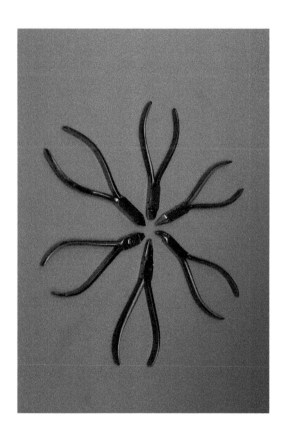

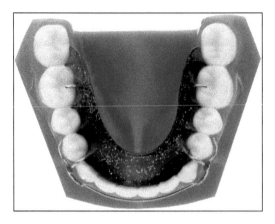

Figure 16.1

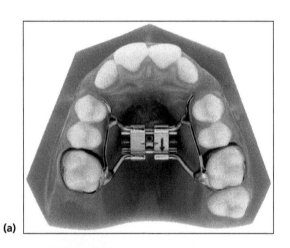

(a)

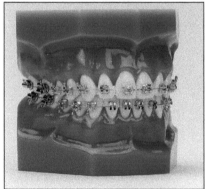

(b)

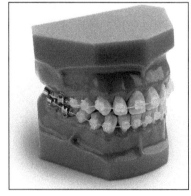

(c)

Figure 16.2

ORTHODONTIC INSTRUMENTS

ORTHODONTIC APPLIANCES

FIGURE 16.1

Name
Removable orthodontic appliance (Hawley retainer)

Features
- Is removable and depends on patient compliance for success
- Constructed from acrylic and a combination of stainless steel retentive clasps and springs
- The acrylic of a removable appliance can be adjusted by grinding with a straight handpiece and acrylic bur, and the clasps and spring can be adjusted with a variety of orthodontic pliers

Varieties
There are many types of removable appliances depending on the needs of the patient (e.g. expansion appliances and Hawley retainers)

FIGURE 16.2a, b, c

Name
Fixed orthodontic appliances: (a) Rapid palatal expander (b) Metal fixed appliance (c) Ceramic fixed appliance

Features
- Are cemented to the teeth and cannot be removed by the patient
- Consist of a combination of orthodontic bands, orthodontic brackets or orthodontic wires
- Require special orthodontic pliers for adjustments

Varieties
There are many types of fixed appliances depending on the needs of the patient (e.g. braces and palatal expanders)

ORTHODONTIC INSTRUMENTS

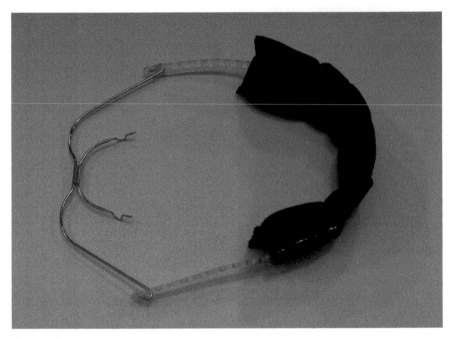

Figure 16.3

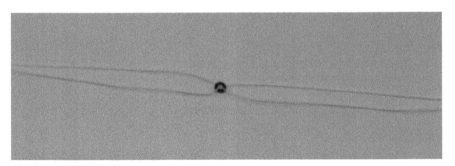

Figure 16.4

ORTHODONTIC INSTRUMENTS

FIGURE 16.3

Name
Headgear and face bow

Function and features
- Has an inner bow (fits into the buccal tubes of the fixed appliance) soldered to an outer bow (can be attached to a strap)
- The headgear is worn outside the mouth, and the face bow is attached to the buccal tubes intra-orally
- The orthodontic headgear is used to prevent establishment of deep overbites by restricting the growth of the maxillary arch. Can also be used to prevent mesial drifting of maxillary molars when teeth have been extracted anterior to the molars
- The strap has a safety mechanism which prevents the bow from springing back at the patient if it is pulled forwards

Varieties
Different sizes available colour coded

ORTHODONTIC MATERIALS

FIGURE 16.4

Name
Elastic separators

Function and placement
- Used to create inter-proximal space to allow orthodontic bands to be placed
- Separators can be placed with floss or separator placing pliers (see Figure 6.11)

ORTHODONTIC INSTRUMENTS

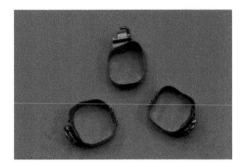

Figure 16.5

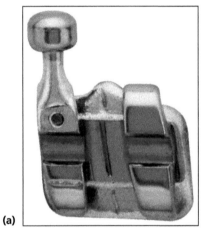

(a)

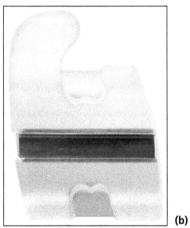

(b)

Figure 16.6

FIGURE 16.5

Name
Orthodontic band

Function, features and placement
- Used to secure auxiliary devices to aid in tooth positioning
- Stainless steel bands are cemented on posterior teeth
- Pre-formed – variety of sizes available
- Occlusal edge is slightly rounded, whereas gingival edge is straight
- Placement is preceded by placement of separators to create interproximal space

Varieties
Available in different shapes and sizes

FIGURE 16.6a, b

Name
(a) Metal orthodontic bracket (b) Ceramic orthodontic bracket

Function and features
- Used to secure an orthodontic archwire in place
- Most often bonded to the buccal surface of the tooth
- Orthodontic brackets may have coloured indicators to help orientate placement
- Orthodontic brackets often have a textured back that aids in bonding to the tooth

Varieties
- Many different brands and sizes available
- Can be made from different materials (e.g. stainless steel and ceramics)

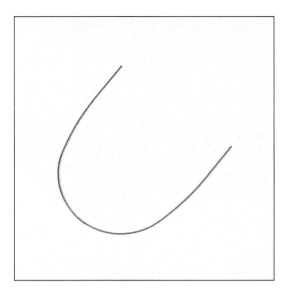

Figure 16.7

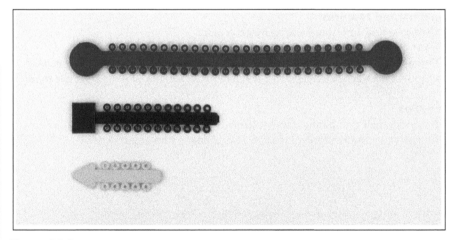

Figure 16.8

ORTHODONTIC INSTRUMENTS

FIGURE 16.7

Name
- Orthodontic archwire

Function and mechanism of action
- Archwires are tied into orthodontic brackets that have been previously bonded to teeth, and these act as a track to facilitate movement of teeth
- The archwire is pre-formed. When tied into the bracket its shape may be altered. This results in force being applied to the teeth as the archwire tries to regain its original shape

Varieties
- Available in different shapes and diameters
- Made from many different materials, e.g. stainless steel and nickel titanium

FIGURE 16.8

Name
Elastomeric modules

Function and directions for use
- Used to ligate or hold the orthodontic archwire in place
- Used with mosquito artery forceps or Mathieu ligature pliers to place around orthodontic brackets
- One use and changed each time the archwire is changed

Varieties
- Can be made from a variety of materials
- Available in many colours

ORTHODONTIC INSTRUMENTS

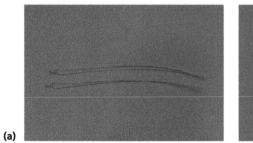 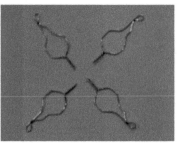

(a)   **(b)**

Figure 16.9

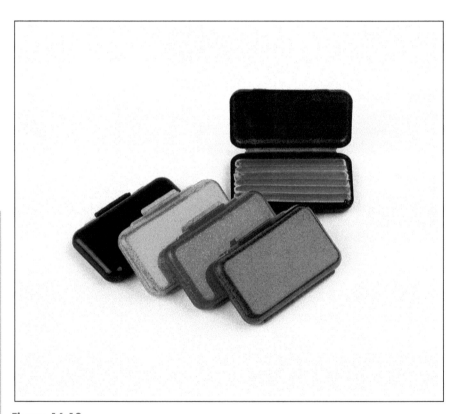

Figure 16.10

FIGURE 16.9a, b

Name
Ligatures

Function and directions for use
- Used to ligate or hold the orthodontic archwire in place
- Used with mosquito artery forceps or Mathieu ligature pliers to place around orthodontic brackets
- Changed each time the archwire is changed
- The excess ligature wire is cut with various orthodontic pliers and should be disposed of in the sharps' bin
- One use

Varieties
- Can be made from a variety of materials
- Different types: (a) long ligature, (b) 'quick ligs' and Kobayashi tie hooks that facilitate tying elastics around

FIGURE 16.10

Name
Patient relief wax (bee's wax)

Function
Given to the patient after fixed appliance placement to help relieve discomfort from tissue trauma

ORTHODONTIC INSTRUMENTS

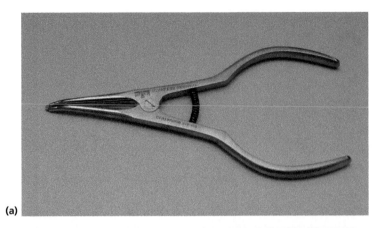

(a)

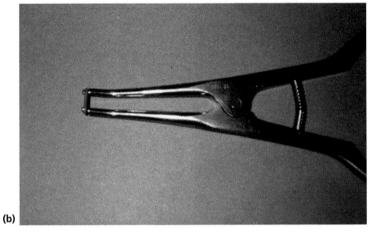

(b)

Figure 16.11

ORTHODONTIC INSTRUMENTS

FIGURE 16.11a, b

Name
Separator placing pliers

Function and features
• Used for placing elastic separators interproximally
• Single-ended instrument – handle is adapted for a palm grasp

Varieties
Different sizes and shapes are available

False friends
Rubber dam clamp forceps and Coons ligature pliers

FIGURE 16.12

Name
Johnson contouring pliers

Function and features
• Used to re-contour and adapt an orthodontic band to a tooth
• Beaks are tapered with a slight bow
• One beak is concave while the other is convex allowing re-contouring of bands

Varieties
Shape of beaks may vary

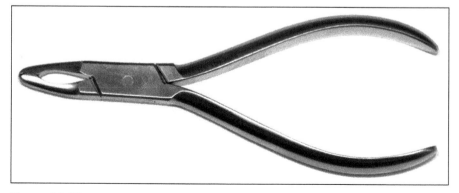

Figure 16.12

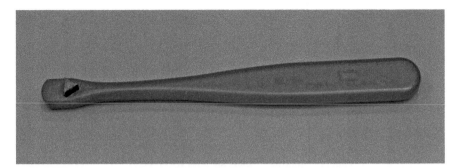

Figure 16.13

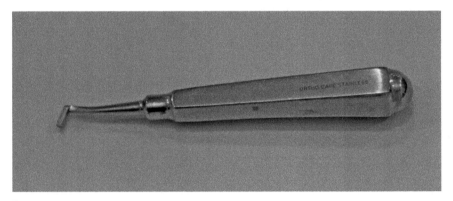

Figure 16.14

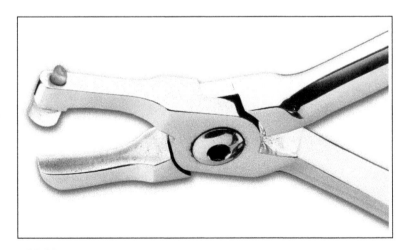

Figure 16.15

ORTHODONTIC INSTRUMENTS

FIGURE 16.13

Name
Nylon band seater

Function and features
- Used for the patient to bite to facilitate the seating of an orthodontic band
- Edge of the tip is serrated to facilitate grip
- Autoclavable

Varieties
Many shapes and sizes available

FIGURE 16.14

Name
Mershon band pusher

Functions and features
- Aid in the placement and seating of orthodontic bands
- Can be used to adapt the coronal portion of the band to the tooth
- Handle is designed to allow better operator grasp

False friend
Couplands chisel

FIGURE 16.15

Name
Posterior band remover

Function, features and method of use
- Used to remove posterior orthodontic bands
- Two stainless steel beaks, one may have a nylon tip (may be replaceable)
- When removing a band, the nylon tip is placed on the occlusal surface, and the curved beak is placed at the gingival edge of the band

Varieties
- Different sizes and shapes available
- Tip may be metal instead of nylon

ORTHODONTIC INSTRUMENTS

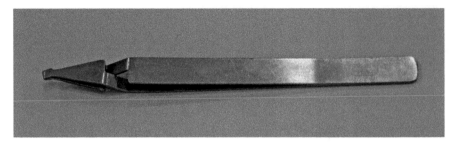

Figure 16.16

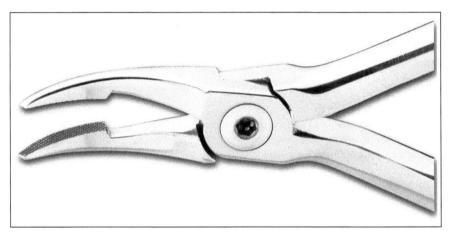

Figure 16.17

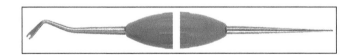

Figure 16.18

FIGURE 16.16

Name
Bracket holder

Function
- Securely grasps the orthodontic bracket during placement
- Applying pressure opens working end and releasing closes working end

Varieties
- Different sizes and shapes available
- Control mechanism may vary

FIGURE 16.17

Name
Weingart pliers

Functions and feature
- Used to guide and move the archwire in and out of placement
- Used to hold the archwire during bending
- The bend in the beak facilitates easy grasping of the archwire and guiding into buccal tubes

Varieties
Different shapes and sizes of beaks available

FIGURE 16.18

Name
Ligature tucker/ligature director

Function and feature
- Used to tuck excess ligature wire out of the way to reduce tissue trauma
- Notch in working end allows operator to apply pressure to archwire to bend it into place

Varieties
- Can be single-ended or double-ended
- Different sizes and shapes of working ends

ORTHODONTIC INSTRUMENTS

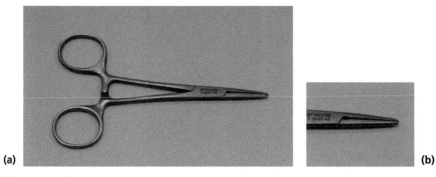

(a)   (b)

Figure 16.19

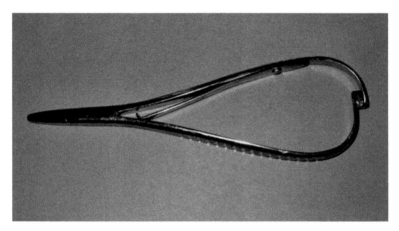

Figure 16.20

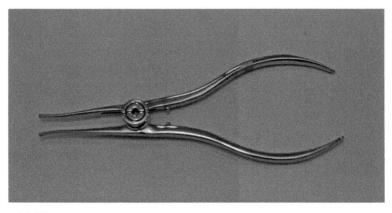

Figure 16.21

FIGURE 16.19a, b

Name
Mosquito artery forceps – straight

Function and feature
- Used to grasp and place orthodontic separators, power chain and modules
- Beak is serrated for better grasp

Varieties
Different sizes and shapes are available

False friends
Beebee crown scissors/shears, needle holders

FIGURE 16.20

Name
Mathieu ligature pliers

Function and features
- Used to grasp and place ligature wires and elastics
- Beaks are serrated for better grasp
- The handle has a locking mechanism and a spring mechanism that help the operator to quickly open and close the pliers

Varieties
Beaks can vary in length and angle

FIGURE 16.21

Name
Coon's ligature pliers

Function
Used to tie long ligatures into a 'figure-of-eight'

Varieties
Various angles and sizes of beaks

False friends
Rubber dam clamp forceps and separator placing pliers

ORTHODONTIC INSTRUMENTS

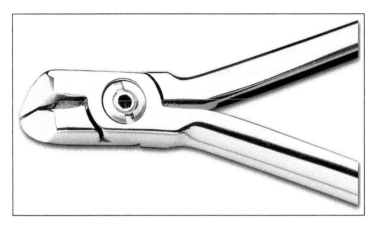

Figure 16.22

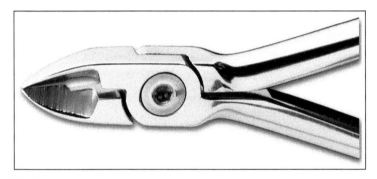

Figure 16.23

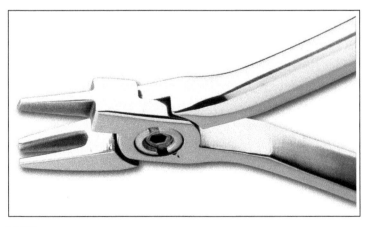

Figure 16.24

FIGURE 16.22

Name
Distal end cutter

Function and features
- Used to cut the distal portion of an orthodontic archwire
- Can be used extra-orally (prior to placement)
- Can be used intra-orally (after placement)
- There is a 'safety' mechanism to hold the cut archwire so it does not fall into the patients mouth

Varieties
Various angles and sizes of beaks

FIGURE 16.23

Name
Ligature cutter

Function and features
- Used to cut ligature wires (not to be used on ligatures more than 0.015 mm in diameter as it damages the cutting edge)
- Can also be used to cut elastics and power chains
- Edges are sharp and can be sharpened when they become dull

Varieties
- Variety of beaks and cutting angles
- Some may have replaceable beaks

FIGURE 16.24

Name
Triple beak pliers

Functions
- Used to place a bend in an orthodontic archwire
- Used to contour and shape an orthodontic archwire

Varieties
Beaks may vary in size and shape

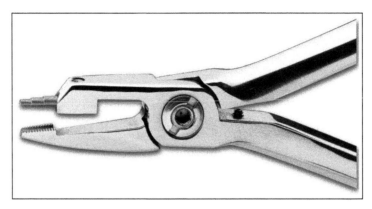

Figure 16.25

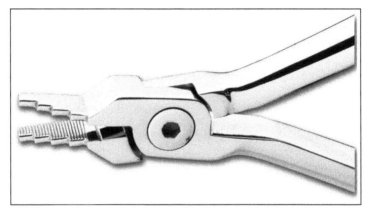

Figure 16.26

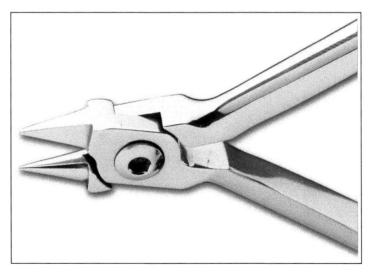

Figure 16.27

ORTHODONTIC INSTRUMENTS

FIGURE 16.25

Name
Omega pliers

Function and feature
- Used to bend and form loops in orthodontic archwires
- Grooves in beaks facilitate bending loops into archwires
- Used to bend removable appliance wires

Varieties
Beaks may vary in size and shape

FIGURE 16.26

Name
Nance pliers

Function
Used to hold and bend orthodontic archwires

Varieties
Beaks may vary depending on the type of archwire to be bent

FIGURE 16.27

Name
Light wire pliers

Function
Used to bend and place loops in an orthodontic archwire

Varieties
Variety of beaks

False friend
Adams spring forming pliers

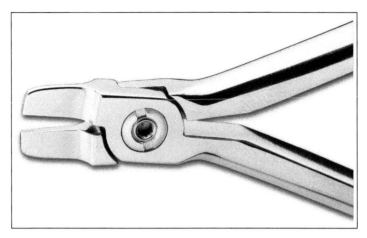

Figure 16.28

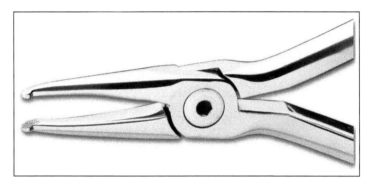

Figure 16.29

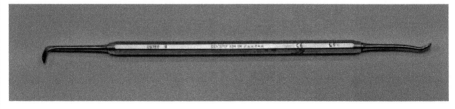

Figure 16.30

FIGURE 16.28

Name
Tweed pliers

Function and feature
- Used to bend and form loops in orthodontic archwires
- Grooves in beaks facilitate bending loops into archwires

FIGURE 16.29

Name
How(e) pliers

Functions and features
- Multipurpose orthodontic pliers
- A long beak with serrated tips for grasping
- Can be used to grasp bands and archwires during placement and removal, and to tie metal ligatures

Varieties
Beaks may vary in size and shape

FIGURE 16.30

Name
Mitchell trimmer

Functions
- Used after placement of orthodontic bands to remove excess cement
- Can be used after de-bonding brackets in the removal of excess cement with a conventional handpiece and a de-bonding bur

False friends
Hollenback $3^{1}/_{2}$ carver, Wards carver

ORTHODONTIC INSTRUMENTS

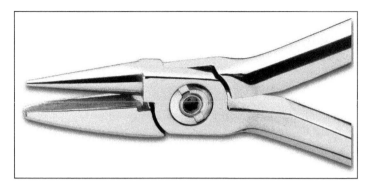

Figure 16.31

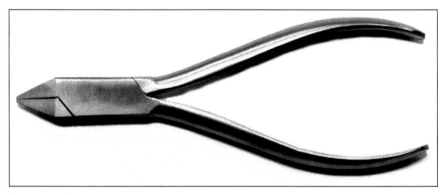

Figure 16.32

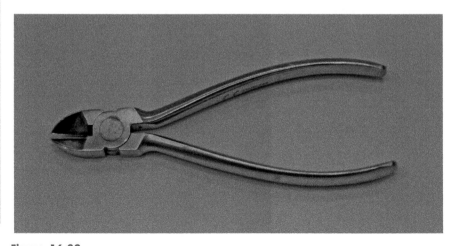

Figure 16.33

FIGURE 16.31

Name
Adams spring forming pliers

Functions and features
- Used to adjust springs on orthodontic removable appliances
- Can be used to smooth and contour archwires
- One beak is rounded, the other is square/flat ended

Varieties
- Beaks may vary in size and shape

False friend
Light wire pliers

FIGURE 16.32

Name
Adams universal pliers

Function
Used to adjust headgear, face bows and Adams clasps on removable appliances

Varieties
Different sizes are available

False friend
Adams spring forming pliers

FIGURE 16.33

Name
Mauns heavy duty wire cutter

Function
To cut heavy archwires or appliance wires – used extra-orally

Varieties
Different sizes and shapes of beaks are available

ORTHODONTIC INSTRUMENTS

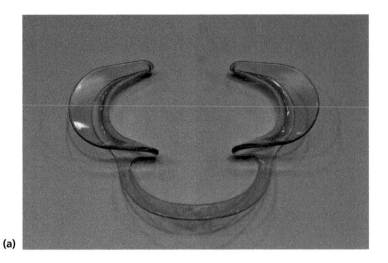

(a)

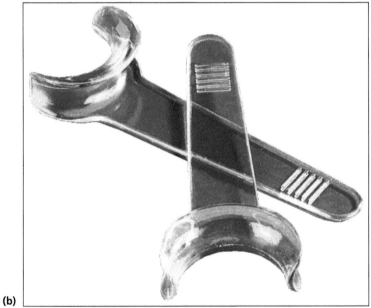

(b)

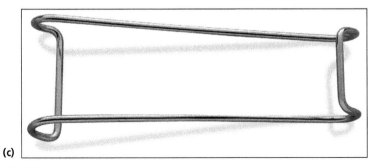

(c)

Figure 16.34

MISCELLANEOUS ITEMS

FIGURE 16.34a, b, c

Name

Cheek retractors

Functions

- To retract cheeks and lips for better visibility
- Often used when bonding fixed appliances and taking photographs

Varieties

- Different sizes and shapes available
- Plastic and metal types available

FIGURE 16.35

Name

Intra-oral mirrors

Function

- Aid in visibility when taking intra-oral photographs
- Often used in conjunction with cheek retractors

Varieties

Different sizes and shapes available

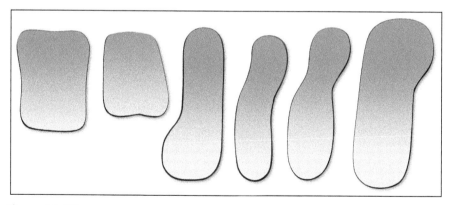

Figure 16.35

ORTHODONTIC INSTRUMENTS

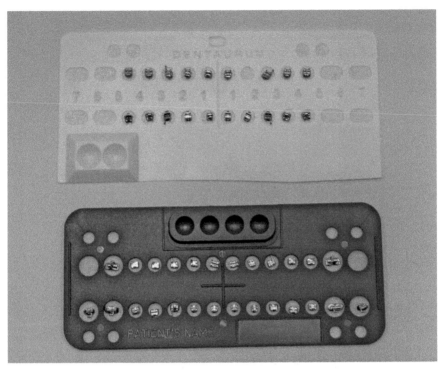

Figure 16.36

FIGURE 16.36

Name
Orthodontic bracket card

Function and features
- Used to organise and hold orthodontic brackets to facilitate quick bracket placement
- Each circle on the card corresponds to a particular tooth in the mouth
- Brackets are placed corresponding to the tooth to be bonded
- Tape on the back of the card helps to keep brackets in place

ORTHODONTIC INSTRUMENTS

Set-ups

The following instruments are common to all the below listed set-ups:
- Mouth mirror and handle (p. 34, 35)
- Sickle/contra-angled probe (p. 36, 37)
- College tweezers (p. 39, 40)
- Hand mirror

Separator placement
- Dental floss
- Elastomeric separators
- Separator placing pliers

Band placement
- (Separators placed one week in advance of this appointment)
- Orthodontic bands
- High volume suction (p. 42, 43)
- Low volume suction/saliva ejector (p. 42, 43)
- Prophy handpiece (p. 74, 75)
- Rubber cup (p. 84, 85)
- Pumice
- Orthodontic bands
- Mershon band pusher
- Contouring pliers
- Posterior band remover
- Nylon band seater
- Cotton wool rolls (p. 44, 45)
- Glass ionomer cement
- Weston spatula (p. 92, 93)
- Mitchell trimmer
- Air/water syringe/3-in-1 syringes (p. 46, 47)

Bracket placement
- Instructions for care of new fixed appliance
- Orthodontic brackets, bands, archwire, elastics, power chain and ligatures
- High volume suction, low volume suction/disposable saliva ejector (p. 42, 43)
- Air/water syringe/3-in-1 syringe (p. 46, 47)
- Prophy handpiece, prophy cup and flour of pumice (pp. 74 and 75)
- Cheek retractors (p. 174–176)
- Acid etch
- Bonding agent
- Dappen dish (p. 94, 95)
- Composite gun (p. 102, 103)
- Composite (p. 102, 103)
- Curing light (p. 108, 109)
- Teflon-tipped flat plastic (p. 105, 106)
- Bracket holders

- Orthodontic archwire
- Ligature tucker
- Ligature cutter
- Distal end cutter
- Mosquito artery forceps
- Elastomeric modules
- Ligatures
- Johnson contouring pliers, Weingart, Tweed and triple beak pliers – depending on operator's preference

Archwire change
- Weingart pliers
- Distal end cutter
- Ligature tucker
- Ligature cutter

De-bond, fixed appliance removal
- Posterior band remover
- Conventional handpiece and de-bonding bur
- Mitchell trimmer
- How(e) pliers
- Posterior band remover

If patient will need a removable appliance
- Impression materials
- Impression trays, adhesive, mixing spatula, mixing bowl and water measure (p. 213)
- Laboratory prescription and bag

Delivery of removable appliance
- Straight handpiece
- Acrylic burs
- Adams pliers
- Mauns heavy duty wire cutter
- Appliance box
- Instructions on care of new appliance
- Hand mirror

Appliance adjustment
- Straight handpiece (p. 72, 73)
- Acrylic burs (p. 78, 79)
- Adams universal pliers
- Adams spring forming pliers
- Mauns heavy duty wire cutter
- Miller's forceps (p. 110, 111)
- Articulating paper (p. 110, 111)

SECTION 17
INSTRUMENTS USED IN PERIODONTAL PROCEDURES

Maintenance of the health of the periodontium (gingiva, periodontal ligament and alveolar bone) is vital for an individual's overall dental health. Disease of the periodontium is referred to as periodontal disease and is a common dental problem. The dental team uses specialised instruments to maintain good periodontal health or to reverse the effects of periodontal disease.

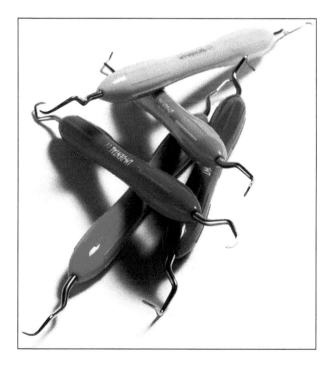

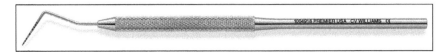

Figure 17.1

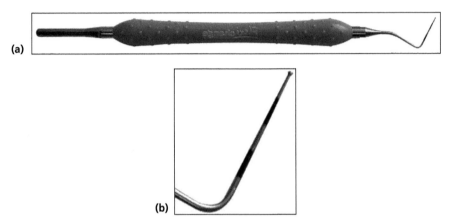

(a)

(b)

Figure 17.2

VARIOUS PERIODONTAL PROBES

FIGURE 17.1

Name
Williams periodontal probe

Function and feature
- Used to probe the depth of a periodontal pocket, allowing the operator to measure the pocket depth by reading the markings
- Working end is marked in millimetres to measure periodontal pockets around teeth (can probe depths as small as 0.4 mm)

Varieties
- Can be single-ended or double-ended
- Many different types of periodontal probes available

False friends
Endodontic probe (DG16 probe), endodontic spreader, BPE/CPITN probe (BPE, basic periodontal examination; CPITN, community periodontal index of treatment needs)

FIGURE 17.2a, b

Name
BPE/CPITN probe

Function and features
- Ball on working end helps to prevent tissue trauma and detect sub-gingival calculus
- The coloured bands are for measuring the depth of periodontal pockets
- The measurements recorded will indicate to the operator the level of periodontal treatment needed
- Calibrated in millimetres

False friend
Periodontal probe

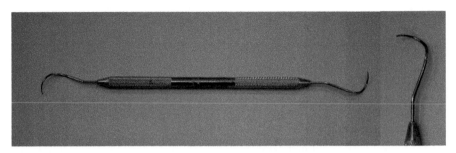

Figure 17.3

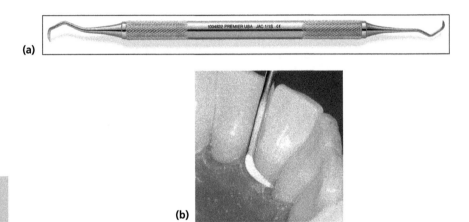

(a)

(b)

Figure 17.4

FIGURE 17.3

Name
Furcation probe

Functions and features
- To examine tooth surfaces and detect imperfections in furcations, pit, fissures, inter-proximal areas and around restorations
- Measures the depth of furcation involvement
- There is a pointed working end calibrated in millimetres (denoted by black markings)

Varieties
- Can be single-ended or double-ended
- Variety of working ends

SCALERS AND CURETTES

FIGURE 17.4a, b

Name
Jacquette scaler

Function, features and method of use
- Used with a pull action
- To remove supra-gingival calculus and plaque
- Two cutting edges that meet at a point
- Needs to be sharpened regularly

Varieties
- Can be single-ended or double-ended
- Many different types are available

False friends
Gracey curettes

INSTRUMENTS USED IN
PERIODONTAL PROCEDURES

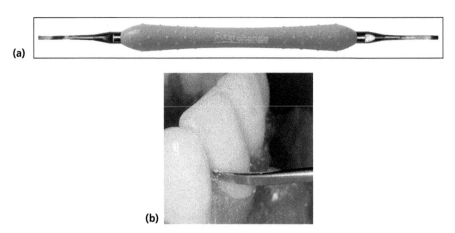

(a)

(b)

Figure 17.5

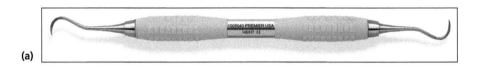

(a)

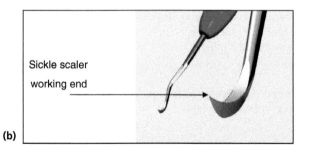

Sickle scaler
working end

(b)

Figure 17.6

FIGURE 17.5a, b

Name
Push scaler

Function and method of use
- Used with a push action
- To remove supra-gingival calculus and plaque

Varieties
Can be single-ended or double-ended

False friends
Enamel chisel, enamel hatchet

FIGURE 17.6a, b

Name
Sickle scaler

Function and features
- To remove supra-gingival calculus and plaque
- Two cutting edges that meet at a point
- Needs to be sharpened regularly

Varieties
- Available as anterior or posterior instruments with a variety of working ends
- Can be single-ended or double-ended

False friends
Sickle/contra-angled probe, Gracey curettes

INSTRUMENTS USED IN
PERIODONTAL PROCEDURES

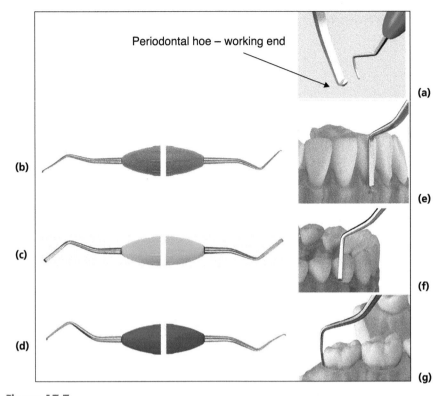

Figure 17.7

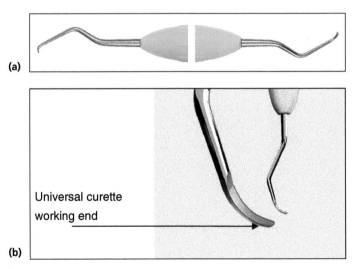

Figure 17.8

FIGURE 17.7a, b, c, d, e, f, g

Name
Periodontal hoes

Function and method of use
- To remove supra-gingival and sub-gingival calculus and plaque
- Used with a push–pull action
- May have tungsten carbide working ends for added strength

Varieties
- Can be available as different types for working in specific areas (anterior, buccal/lingual surfaces and posterior)
- Can be single-ended or double-ended

False friends
Push scaler, enamel chisel

FIGURE 17.8a, b

Name
Universal curette

Function and features
- Used to remove stains, supra-gingival and sub-gingival calculus and plaque, and used in root planing
- Designed to adapt to all areas and surfaces of the mouth
- The working ends are usually mirror images of each other (double-ended instrument) and are perpendicular to the lower shank
- There are two cutting edges that meet at a rounded working end

Varieties
Can be single-ended or double-ended

False friend
Scalers

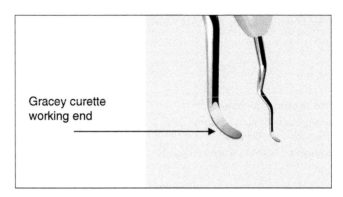

Figure 17.9

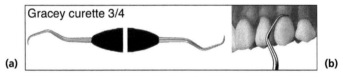

Figure 17.10

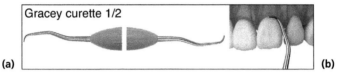

Figure 17.11

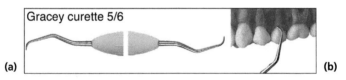

Figure 17.12

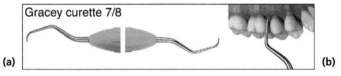

Figure 17.13

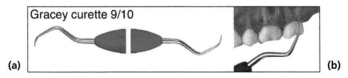

Figure 17.14

FIGURES 17.9; 17.10a, b; 17.11a, b; 17.12a, b; 17.13a, b; 17.14a, b; 17.15a, b; 17.16a, b

Name
Gracey curettes

Function and features
- Designed to adapt to specific areas in the mouth
- An operator will need a full set of instruments to work in all areas of the mouth
- Have one cutting edge and a rounded working end
- Used to remove stains, sub-gingival calculus and for root planing
- The name of the instrument consists of a name (usually indicating the person, institution, etc., who designed the instrument) followed by two numbers (if the instrument is double-ended) that refer to the working ends
- If the instrument has two numbers on the handle, each number refers to the working end that it is closest to
- The number indicates the specific area the Gracey curette will be used in:
  - Gracey 1/2, 3/4 (Figures 17.10, 17.11) – incisors and canines
  - Gracey 5/6 (Figure 17.12) – premolars
  - Gracey 7/8, 9/10 (Figures 17.13, 17.14) – buccal and lingual surfaces of the posterior teeth
  - Gracey 11/12 (Figure 17.15) – mesial surfaces of posterior teeth
  - Gracey 13/14 (Figure 17.16) – distal surfaces of posterior teeth
- Need to be sharpened regularly with a sharpening stone, or they can be professionally sharpened

Varieties
- Many types of curettes are available (mini, macro, standard and rigid Gracey curettes)
- Can be single-ended or double-ended

False friends
Scalers

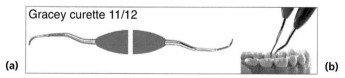

(a)   (b)

Figure 17.15

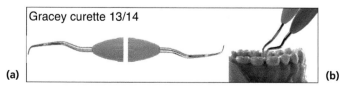

(a)   (b)

Figure 17.16

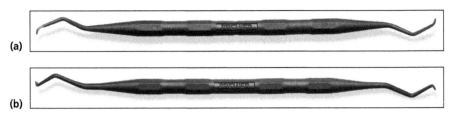

Figure 17.17

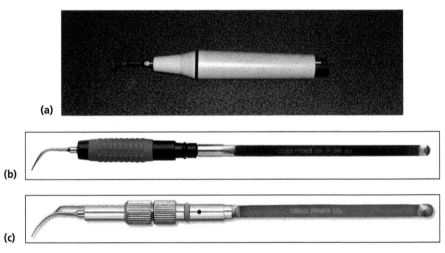

Figure 17.18

FIGURE 17.17a, b

Name
Implant scalers

Function and feature
- Used to remove plaque, calculus and stains from implants
- Designed so as not to cause damage to or scratch the implant
- Available with gold-tipped working end or plastic so the implant will not be damaged or scratched

Varieties
Many different sizes and shapes available

FIGURE 17.18a, b, c

Name
Ultrasonic scaler tips

Function and features
- Used in conjunction with an ultrasonic scaling unit to remove stains, plaque and calculus (using ultrasonic waves)
- Water is used with this instrument
- Handle fits on the dental unit
- The ultrasonic tips are interchangeable

Varieties
- Different tips are available depending on use, e.g. sub-gingival and universal
- Many different makes and systems available (e.g. Cavitron)

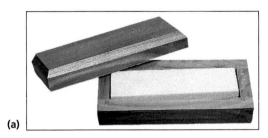
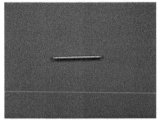

Figure 17.19

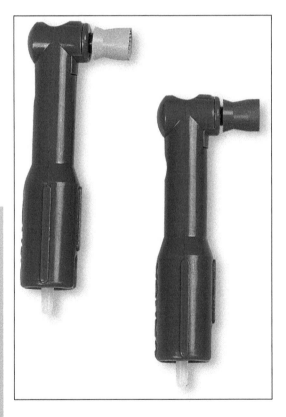

Figure 17.20

MISCELLANEOUS EQUIPMENT

FIGURE 17.19a, b

Name
(a) Sharpening stone (b) Plastic test stick

Functions and importance
- A sharpening stone is used to grind, sharpen and smooth the working ends of sharp hand instruments (can be used with a sharpening oil)
- A sharp instrument facilitates easier removal of deposits, reduces time needed to clean, minimises patient discomfort, improves tactile sensitivity of the operator and reduces hand fatigue for the operator
- A plastic test stick is used to check that the working end is sharp

Varieties
Sharpening stones are available in different grits, sizes and shapes

FIGURE 17.20

Name
Disposable prophy angle attachments (please see Section 7 for conventional handpiece, rubber polishing cups and bristle brush)

Function and features
- Used to polish teeth
- Single use
- Designed for infection control purposes
- Attach to conventional handpiece

Varieties
Many different sizes and shapes available

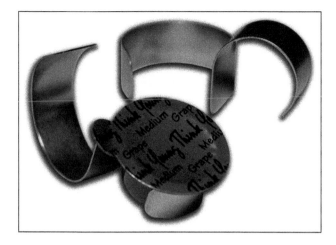

Figure 17.21

FIGURE 17.21

Name
Prophy ring

Function
Used to hold unidose prophy paste during rubber cup polishing

Varieties
Various sizes and shapes available from different manufacturers

INSTRUMENTS USED IN
PERIODONTAL PROCEDURES

Set-ups

The following instruments are common to all the below listed set-ups:
- Mouth mirror and handle (p. 34, 35)
- Periodontal probe (p. 36, 37)
- Sickle/contra-angled probe (p. 36, 37)
- College tweezers (p. 39, 40)
- Hand mirror
- Furcation probe

Routine periodontal recall
- Sickle scaler
- Various Gracey curettes
- Arkansas sharpening stone
- Plastic test stick
- Prophy handpiece (p. 74, 75)
- Rubber polishing cup (p. 74, 75)
- Prophy paste and/or flour of pumice

Root planing
- Local anaesthetic set-up if required (see Section 5, p. 49)
- Sickle scaler
- Various Gracey curettes
- Ultrasonic scaler
- Arkansas sharpening stone
- Plastic test stick
- Prophy handpiece (p. 74, 75)
- Rubber polishing cup (p. 74, 75)
- Prophy paste or flour of pumice
- Air/water syringe/3-in-1 syringe (p. 46, 47)
- High-volume suction, low-volume suction/saliva ejector (p. 42, 43)

SECTION 18

INSTRUMENTS USED IN REMOVABLE AND FIXED PROSTHODONTICS

Prosthetic dentistry involves the 'prosthetic' or 'false' replacement of natural teeth. There are two divisions of prosthetic dentistry:
- Fixed prosthodontics: the prostheses cannot be removed by the patient, which includes crowns, bridges, implant restorations, veneers and inlays
- Removable prosthodontics: the prostheses can be removed by the patient, which includes full and partial dentures

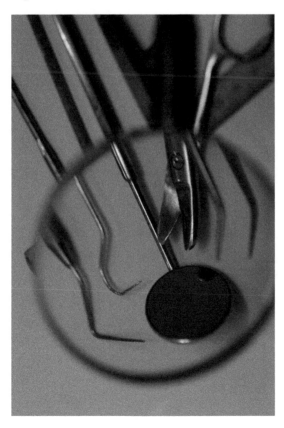

Basic Guide to Dental Instruments, Second Edition. Carmen Scheller-Sheridan.
© 2011 Carmen Scheller-Sheridan. Published 2011 by Blackwell Publishing Ltd.

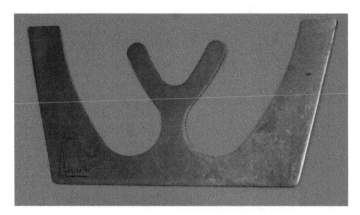

Figure 18.1

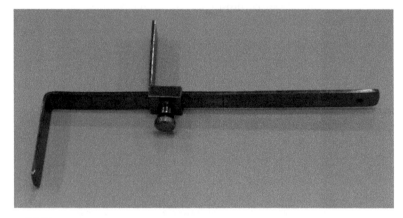

Figure 18.2

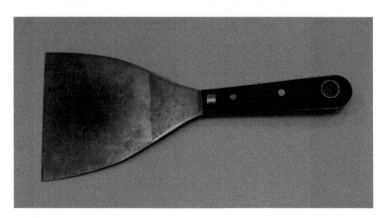

Figure 18.3

FIGURE 18.1

Name
Fox's occlusal plane guide

Functions and indications
- Used with edentulous patients
- Used during the jaw relationship stage of denture construction
- Used to check that the incisal line is in a horizontal plane and that the sides are parallel with a line joining the ala of the nose and the tragus of the ear (the ala-tragal line)
- Always used when the patient is sitting upright

FIGURE 18.2

Name
Willis bite gauge

Function
- Used to measure vertical dimension
- Used during patient assessment and the jaw relationship stage in denture construction

This is how the operator can tell if the edentulous patient's mouth is over-closing or not closing enough during the stage of bite registration

FIGURE 18.3

Name
Paint scraper

Function
Used in conjunction with a heat source to soften and smooth wax rims while recording the patient's occlusion during the jaw relationship stage of denture construction

INSTRUMENTS USED IN REMOVABLE AND FIXED PROSTHODONTICS

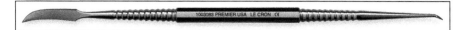

Figure 18.4

(a)

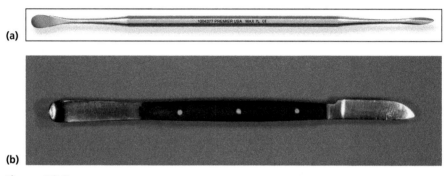

(b)

Figure 18.5

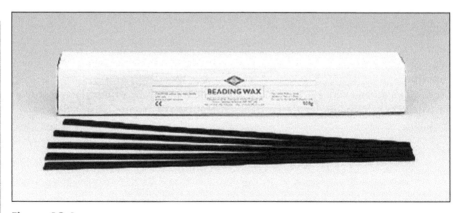

Figure 18.6

FIGURE 18.4

Name
Le Cron carver

Function
Used for fine trimming of wax at various stages of denture construction

False friends
Hollenback $3^{1}/_{2}$ carver, Wards carver, Mitchell trimmer

FIGURE 18.5a, b

Name
Wax knife

Function
For trimming wax during denture construction

FIGURE 18.6

Name
Red ribbon wax

Function
- Used during construction of dentures, crowns and bridges
- Can be used to extend the length or height of impression trays

INSTRUMENTS USED IN REMOVABLE AND FIXED PROSTHODONTICS

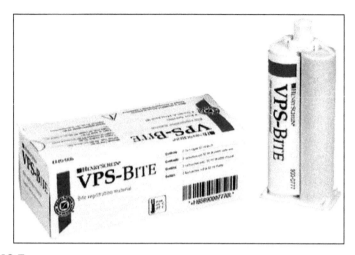

Figure 18.7

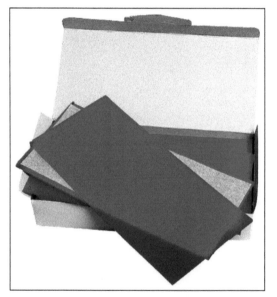

Figure 18.8

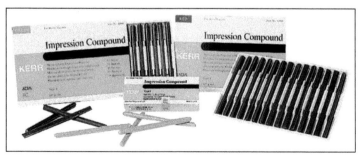

Figure 18.9

FIGURE 18.7

Name
Bite registration paste

Function
Used in conjunction with wax rims to record a patient's occlusal relationship

Varieties
Available in different types and thicknesses

FIGURE 18.8

Name
Modelling wax

Function and method of use
- Used to record a jaw relationship
- May be softened under warm water or used in conjunction with a heat source

Varieties
Available in different types and thicknesses

FIGURE 18.9

Name
Greenstick composition

Function
Heated and softened to extend the periphery of an impression tray, commonly used for border moulding

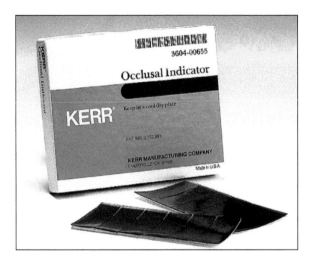

Figure 18.10

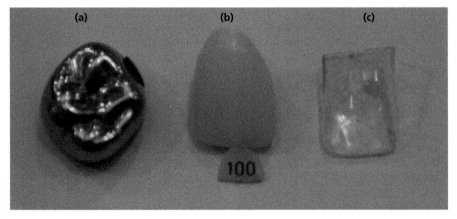

Figure 18.11

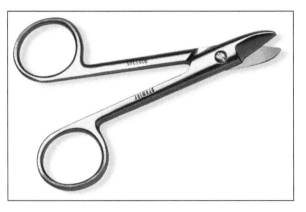

Figure 18.12

FIGURE 18.10

Name
Green occlusal indicating wax

Function
To check the occlusal relationship of upper and lower teeth

Varieties
Available in different delivery systems

FIGURE 18.11a, b, c

Name
Crown forms:

(a) Stainless steel crown form
(b) Polycarbonate crown form
(c) Acetate/clear crown form (celluloid)

Functions
- Used as temporary/provisional crowns during permanent crown fabrication
- Protect the prepared tooth from trauma and sensitivity
- Help to prevent drifting and maintains occlusion with other teeth
- Aesthetically pleasing
- Cemented with a temporary cement

Varieties
Available in different sizes and shapes

FIGURE 18.12

Name
Beebee crown scissors/shears

Function
Cutting and trimming various materials, e.g. rubber dam septa and provisional/temporary crowns

Varieties
Various shapes and sizes are available

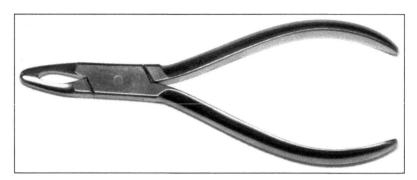

Figure 18.13

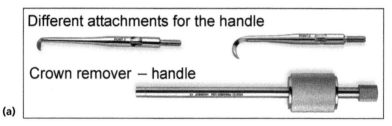

Different attachments for the handle

Crown remover – handle

(a)

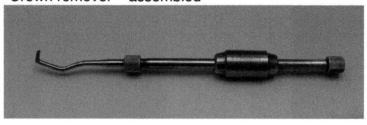

Crown remover – assembled

(b)

Figure 18.14

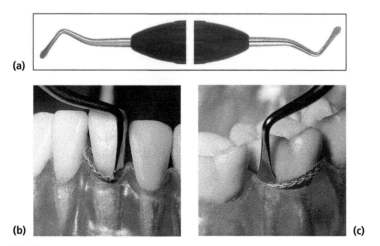

(a)

(b)   **(c)**

Figure 18.15

FIGURE 18.13

Name
Johnson contouring pliers

Function and features
- Used to re-contour and adapt stainless steel crowns
- Beaks are tapered with a slight bow
- One beak is concave and the other is convex for re-contouring crowns

Varieties
Shapes of beaks may vary

FIGURE 18.14a, b

Name
Crown remover

Function and method of use
- Used to remove cemented crowns
- Beak of instrument is placed at the gingival margin of the crown while the weight on the handle is lightly tapped
- The light tapping may result in enough force to remove the crown

FIGURE 18.15a, b, c

Name
Cord packer/gingival retraction cord instrument

Functions
- Used to 'pack' gingival retraction cord into the sulcus prior to taking a final impression
- Can be used to retract tissues if access to a restoration is limited

Varieties
Working ends are available in many different sizes and shapes

INSTRUMENTS USED IN REMOVABLE AND FIXED PROSTHODONTICS

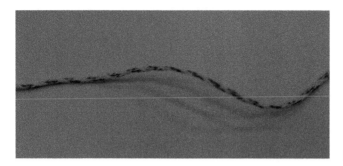

Figure 18.16

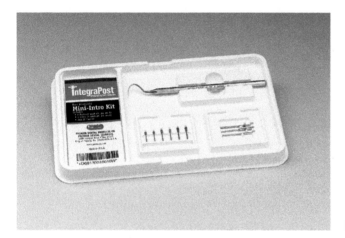

Figure 18.17

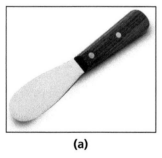

(a)

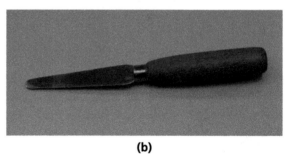

(b)

Figure 18.18

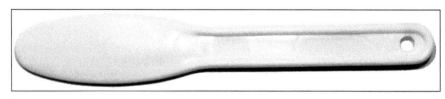

Figure 18.19

FIGURE 18.16

Name
Gingival retraction cord

Function and direction for use
- Packed into the gingival sulcus to retract the gingiva, to get an accurate impression of the prepared crown margins
- Can be soaked in a haemostatic agent to control bleeding as most impression materials are moisture sensitive

Varieties
Available in different thicknesses, in single dose packets or a strand that must be cut to required size

FIGURE 18.17

Name
Pre-fabricated/pre-formed post-kit

Function and kit contents
- Used after root canal treatment to help retain the build-up on the tooth
- The kit contains post-drills and pre-fabricated posts

Varieties
- Many different types available
- Cast posts can be fabricated where indicated

FIGURE 18.18a, b

Name
Wooden-handled impression spatulas

Function
For mixing impression materials

FIGURE 18.19

Name
Fish-tail spatula

Function
For mixing alginate impression materials

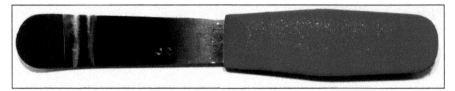

Figure 18.20

FIGURE 18.20

Name
Plaster spatula

Function
For mixing plaster and stone materials

Set-ups

Fixed Prosthodontics

(Note: Many instruments listed here may be illustrated in other sections due to their multiple functions.)

The following instruments are common to all the below listed set-ups:
- Mouth mirror and handle (p. 34, 35)
- Sickle/contra-angled probe (p. 36, 37)
- College tweezers (p. 39, 40)
- High and low volume/disposable saliva ejector suction tips (p. 42, 43)
- Cotton wool rolls (p. 44, 45)
- Local anaesthetic set-up (see Section 5, p. 49)
- Floss
- Miller forceps and articulating paper (p. 110, 111)

Inlays, crowns and bridges
First visit:
- Turbine handpiece and burs (see Section 7, p. 69)
- Conventional handpiece and burs (see Section 7, p. 69)
- Mandrels and discs (p. 82, 83)
- Impression materials, impression trays and adhesive material (opposing arch impression; see Section 15, p. 213)
- If a restoration is needed – see set-up in Section 8, p. 87
- Temporary filling material or temporary/provisional crown or bridge material
- Laboratory prescription and laboratory bag
- Method for disinfection prior to sending to the laboratory
- Shade guide
- Gingival retraction cord
- Flat plastic instrument
- Waxes

Second visit:
- Mosquito artery forceps
- Gauze to protect patient's airway during cementation
- Cement for permanent cementation, e.g. zinc phosphate
- Turbine handpiece and burs (see Section 7, p. 69)
- Conventional handpiece, prophy cup, pumice and burs (see Section 7, p. 69)
- Mixing spatula and paper pad
- Shimstock

Removable Prosthodontics

The following instruments are common to all the below listed set-ups:
- Mouth mirror and handle (p. 34, 35)
- Sickle/contra-angled probe (p. 36, 37)
- College tweezers (p. 39, 40)

INSTRUMENTS USED IN REMOVABLE AND FIXED PROSTHODONTICS

- Ball burnisher (p. 98, 99)
- Bowl of water to keep old denture moist
- Method for disinfection prior to sending to the laboratory

Denture fabrication: (if the construction is for replacement of dentures, a soft reline may be needed to restore tissue health)

First visit:
- Impression materials, impression trays and adhesive material
- Willis bite gauge
- Laboratory prescription and laboratory bag
- Shade guide

Second visit:
- Custom trays/special trays (made by the laboratory) (p. 215, 216)
- Impression materials, impression trays and adhesive material
- Laboratory prescription and laboratory bag

Third visit:
- Wax rims (made by laboratory)
- Fox occlusal plane guide
- Paint scraper
- Heat source
- Le Cron carver
- Wax knife
- Bite registration paste
- Laboratory prescription and laboratory bag

Fourth visit:
- Denture teeth set in wax try-in (made by laboratory)
- Le Cron carver
- Wax knife
- Fox occlusal plane guide
- Laboratory prescription and laboratory bag
- Hand mirror

Fifth visit:
- Final dentures – fitting (made by laboratory)
- Straight handpiece and acrylic burs (see Section 7, p. 72, 73)
- Pressure-indicating paste
- Miller forceps and articulating paper (p. 110, 111)
- Instructions on home care and a box for the new denture

Basic Guide to Dental Instruments, Second Edition. Carmen Scheller-Sheridan.
© 2011 Carmen Scheller-Sheridan. Published 2011 by Blackwell Publishing Ltd.